ANATOMY OF A SUPER NURSE

The Ultimate Guide to Becoming Nursey

by Kati Kleber, BSN, RN, CCRN

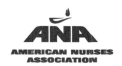

American Nurses Association
Silver Spring, Maryland
2017

This book is about my personal nursing experiences and does not reflect the views of any past or current employers, coworkers, patients, or their loved ones. This book is for informational purposes only. Always refer to your institution's policies, protocols, procedures, as well as your respective state board of nursing and the Standards of Care, and the American Nurses Associations Code of Ethics, as that should be the guiding force behind your practice. The information provided in this book is meant to supplement—not replace—your existing knowledge. Patient stories are discussed; however, multiple identifying details have been changed to protect their privacy and remain compliant with the Health Insurance and Accountability Act of 1996.

American Nurses Association
8515 Georgia Avenue, Suite 400
Silver Spring, MD 20910-3492
1-800-274-4ANA
http://www.NursingWorld.org

The America Nurses Association (ANA) is the premier organization representing the interests of the nation's 3.6 million registered nurses. ANA advances the nursing profession by fostering high standards of nursing practice, promoting a safe and ethical work environment, bolstering the health and wellness of nurses, and advocating on health care issues that affect nurses and the public. ANA is at the forefront of improving the quality of health care for all.

The opinions in this book reflect those of the authors and do not necessarily reflect positions or policies of the American Nurses Association (ANA).

Library of Congress Cataloging-in-Publication Data
Names: Kleber, Kati, author. | American Nurses Association, issuing body.
Title: Anatomy of a super nurse : the ultimate guide to becoming nursey / by Kati Kleber.
Description: [Silver Spring] : American Nurses Association, [2017] | Includes bibliographical references.
Identifiers: LCCN 2017018346 (print) | LCCN 2017018973 (ebook) | ISBN 9781558106925 (ePDF) | ISBN 9781558106932 (ePub) | ISBN 9781558106949 (kindle) | ISBN 9781558106918 (print)
Subjects: | MESH: Nursing | Vocational Guidance | Nursing Process | Clinical Competence | Philosophy, Nursing | United States
Classification: LCC RT82 (ebook) | LCC RT82 (print) | NLM WY 16 AA1 | DDC 610.7306/9--dc23
LC record available at https://lccn.loc.gov/2017018346

978-1-55810-691-8   print   SAN: 851-3481 06/2017
978-1-55810-692-5   ePDF
978-1-55810-693-2   EPUB
978-1-55810-694-9   Kindle

First printing: June 2017

For Christ

Contents

About the Author

Kati Kleber, BSN, RN, CCRN, graduated from nursing school in 2010 in Iowa. After working on a cardiac step-down unit in the Midwest, she worked in neurocritical care in Charlotte, NC. She was a certified preceptor, obtained her critical care certification, and was named one of the Great 100 Nurses of North Carolina and Nurse of the Year by the Charlotte Business Journal in 2015. She has authored three additional books, hosts a podcast for new nurses, and regularly blogs at FreshRN.com.

Kati's passion is not only for encouraging and educating new graduate nurses, but also for building her relationships with other people and God. She and her husband John have one child, Hannah Joy, and two very handsome rescue dogs. To learn more about Kati, please visit katikleber.com.

Introduction

Before I really dive in, I want to give you a better understanding of who I am and why the heck anyone should listen to what I have to say about becoming a safe and successful nurse.

Who I Am

I have been a bachelor's-prepared registered nurse since 2010. I completed a new graduate residency program during my first year out of school while I was working on a cardiothoracic surgical step-down unit. I had a wonderful preceptor and subsequently became a certified preceptor myself. I then worked in a neurosciences critical care unit with another outstanding preceptor and became a certified preceptor in critical care. I have experience working with nursing students, new graduate nurses, and experienced nurses.

However, when I graduated from nursing school and began my first job as a nurse in a residency program I was completely terrified and ill-prepared. I assumed that after thousands of dollars, countless sleepless nights studying, exams covering hundreds of pages worth of material, and one big scary board exam (the NCLEX®) that I would be an awesome nurse. I thought that somehow I would be able to walk into this new facility and just innately know what to do.

I could not have been more wrong. If you had handed me a feeding tube and told me to insert it on a patient the first day on the job, I would have looked at you like a dog does when you give it a command it doesn't know. Head tilt, eyebrow furrow, and all.

The problem is that there is a big gap between learning theory, being introduced to concepts in school, and being handed a license, and actually doing the work of a nurse. The gap is so large that fifty bariatric hospital beds stretched end-to-end could fit there. Nursing school focuses on teaching you very broad topics, many times barely scratching the surface of very detailed and dense issues, simply because there is not enough time. It also discusses and introduces concepts that you can't really learn the specifics of until you are really in the thick of it and the patients are already your responsibility.

As I mentioned, I was overwhelmed and ill-prepared. I was also terrified that I would hurt a patient out of my ignorance and convinced everyone else knew more; therefore, I felt so incredibly alone. I assumed everyone knew what they were doing except for me. Everyone looked so confident and seemed so ready. The other nursing residents had on better scrubs than me, they answered questions faster than me, and everyone seemed to like them better than me. I unknowingly and unnecessarily isolated myself into a corner of inadequacy.

After the first few weeks of sizing each other up during the nurse residency program, all of the nurse residents started to get to know one another and let our guard down. I then came to a powerful and reassuring realization: no one else knew what they were doing either.

We had gone to different nursing schools—some supposedly better and more prestigious than others—and had all passed the NCLEX, yet we were all in the same boat. We were all scared. We were all unsure of how to do simple procedures, how to manage our time, and how to even talk to the other members of the health care team. Nothing can adequately describe the feeling of relief, support, and belonging when I came to this realization. It was like I was climbing a mountain and couldn't see anything except the next tedious step in front of me, and suddenly I was at the summit, surrounded by a breathtaking view.

Despite finally feeling like I could relate to others, I still didn't know what to do when I clocked in for my shifts. So, what do you do when you don't know how to do something but don't want to admit it? You look it up online. I scoured the internet for useful and practical tips, as well as some general encouragement that would help me feel like I had some sort of grasp on this. I couldn't find much, which frustrated me severely. Some of the things I needed to know were very black and white and incredibly important, yet I couldn't find any relatable, concise, and practical information anywhere.

For example, my nursing education taught when to notify physicians, but not how. They especially didn't explain to me how to do this at 0300 when they were half-asleep. I also learned about delegation, but I didn't learn about how to delegate to nursing assistants who had been working on that particular nursing unit for twenty years. And one of the biggest concepts that I had such a difficult time getting a grasp on was time management. I understood the theory behind it, but no clue how to practically carry it out. While I could find information on these topics online, most of it was the same general, big-picture kind of information that was not sufficient.

Once I finally got my feet under me, gained some confidence, and got to the point where I didn't dread going into work every shift, I started taking notes. Those notes formed the backbone of this book, the list of things I learned on the fly but wished I'd found somewhere during my first days on the job, as well as ways to reach out to other new nurses. My goal is to let you know that, while it's okay to feel scared, you should never feel *alone*. We are all in this together and I want you to feel supported from day one. Nursing is a team sport. I became a player in 2010 and now I'm a coach.

How to Use this Book

This book begins with nursing school and concludes with the completion of your first year as a nurse. Regardless of where you are in your career journey, I highly encourage you to read it once all the way through first, even though some aspects of it may not be applicable to you for quite some time. I say this because these sections may be of some help now, even if you are not currently walking through that particular aspect of your journey yet.

This book is meant to be both a source of reference and encouragement. There may be aspects of it that will not be applicable to you for a few years or some that would have been helpful a few years ago. However, a lot of the advice can be adapted for various stages of professional growth. So I encourage you to highlight, bookmark, and come back to things as they become applicable or when you've had a particularly tough shift.

Acknowledgments

I want to thank each and every patient I have had the honor of caring for during my career. I would also like to thank my former coworkers and managers for supporting me during my transition from graduate nurse to bedside nurse, and then again from step-down nurse to neurocritical care nurse. Thank you for your continuous teaching, support, and faith in the nurse that I could become.

This book would not have come to fruition without the constant encouragement and support from my husband. Thank you for being the Office-quoter, exceptional speller, best friend, steadfast supporter, provider, and godly man that you are every single day of my life.

Thank you to my family, who have supported and encouraged me from the day I said, "I think I want to go to nursing school" to the day I said, "I think I want to publish a book," and for buying the first ten copies of every book I publish.

Thank you to the rest of my family and close friends for their honest opinions, encouragement, and support.

And finally, thank you to those who have supported my writing throughout my career, whether it was on the blog, through social media, in person, or all of the above. I sincerely appreciate your encouragement more than I could ever express. You make me a better writer. You make me a better nurse. You make me a better person.

Chapter 1

Gandalf the Grey, RN

"So, why do you want to be a nurse?"

Are you tired of that question yet? People ask it in nursing school interviews, the first day of class and clinicals, job interviews, on applications, and just in casual conversations. For the first five years of my nursing journey, I didn't have a good answer to that question.

For a passionate nurse, I seemed pretty *not* passionate, huh?

I wasn't one of those people who always knew what they wanted to do with their lives. I didn't know what path to take freshmen year of college and didn't have this burning desire in me to become something specific. I envied those who did. My friends who knew they wanted to be teachers, pilots, CPAs, doctors, and so forth all had a passion for it; nothing else would satisfy their professional urge.

I was very aware of the need to quickly make a decision about the path I was going to take but painfully unaware of which path I wanted to take. With so many options, so much potential debt in front of me, and so little time, I made not a passionate decision but a *practical* decision to go into nursing.

Honestly, this was my thought process: "I like teaching and I like health and medicine, so nursing makes sense, right?" I won't pretend it was more complicated than that. That's all I had to go on. I started taking prerequisites at a junior college and prayed that it was the right decision. I prayed I could even get into nursing school—and that I wouldn't hate it.

Surprisingly enough, I quickly found out that I loved nursing. Learning disease processes, caring for patients, and understanding the "why" behind everything was so intriguing to me. I couldn't get enough. Somehow I got through nursing school. Coffee, prayer, and living in the building literally next door to all of my classes (and therefore waking up approximately eight minutes before each class) were my saving graces.

When I started working at the bedside, I discovered that I had found my passion. Even as a young and naïve nurse just surviving each shift, I was able to have a positive impact on my patients. I discovered that you don't have to be one of those expert nurses with years of experience to take good care of a patient.

The Sides of Nursing

Throughout my experience of becoming a nurse, I discovered that being a good nurse isn't as calculated and automated as I had anticipated. Let me explain.

In order to do the job of a nurse, you have to have an awareness and knowledge of technical things like equipment, computers, medications, diagnoses, conditions, and so forth. These are very essential aspects of providing safe patient care. This is what I call the "black" part of nursing. It is very straightforward. There are correct and incorrect answers.

However, there is another side of nursing, one that is not so straightforward. It's when you can walk into a room and instinctively pick up on the emotional climate. You can tell when you need to be comforting, motivating, supportive, or even silent with your patient. You are able to command respect from your patient and their loved ones while still being soft and gentle. You're able to walk into the room of a patient with a completely different cultural background and still bond with them. You're able to earn the patients' and their families' trust quickly. This is what I call the emotional, creative, and social part of nursing, or the "white" part of nursing.

It's putting them both together that truly makes a good nurse. These nurses know enough technical information, yet they also have enough social awareness and emotional intelligence to make their patients feel safely cared for. I call this being a "grey" nurse.

A nurse who is too worried about the black or technical side will be most concerned with their task list. Their bottom line will be, "What's easiest for me?" While tasks may be completed in a technically safe manner that looks good on paper, one must ask, is the patient truly being taken care of when the nurse does not attend to their emotional and mental needs?

Conversely, a nurse too worried about the white or social and emotional side will be most concerned with ensuring all patients feel cared for. Their bottom line will be, "Do my patients feel like I did a good job?" Their patients may have a feeling of security, but are they really receiving safe care if the nurse does not prioritize their physiological needs and understand the technical side of providing care?

A grey nurse would have a very different bottom line. Their bottom line would be, "What is best for the patient?" If what is best for the patient is getting them a central line, starting parenteral feedings, and prepping them to go to the operating room for yet another surgery despite how unpleasant that is for the patient, they will know how to do it safely while also making the patient feel safe, cared for, and heard.

The Good Grey Nurses

But what does being a grey nurse really look like? Those of you looking to begin nursing school or just starting your nursing school journey have an idea about what this may look like, but it is really hard to quantify and understand. It's not comprised of what many people think make a good nurse.

Like I said, I previously envisioned nursing school like an automated machine. In goes a novice, out comes a good nurse: If you just do the work and get the grades, you're guaranteed to be successful.

However, merely having a nursing license and a job on a good unit doesn't make you a good nurse. Working for thirty years doesn't make you a good nurse, nor does being good at starting IVs or becoming best friends with all of the physicians. And it's not about having a commanding presence and knowing all of the answers to the nine hundred questions you get asked each shift. Just because someone is an informal leader with an authoritative presence does not mean they are a good nurse.

Good grey nurses are the ones who can take on a heavy patient load, be a charge nurse, and still somehow be on time with everything, all while making sure all of the nurses working that day feel supported and led. They're the ones who know when they need to drop everything and be there for a patient during a really rough moment. They're the ones patients request by name. They're the ones you go to first when you have a bad feeling about one of your patients. The ones you see on the schedule when you're walking in and feel relieved that they are there that day with you. They're the ones with whom you and your patients feel *safe*.

Good nurses breathe instinct. They breathe discernment. Good nurses can pick out seemingly insignificant things about a patient, interpret an intricate clinical picture, predict a poor outcome, and bring it to the doctor's attention, literally saving someone's life. Good nurses save lives every single day.

Yes, you read that correctly: A normal day at work for a good nurse includes saving the lives of others.

When you don't work at the bedside—in the trenches, so to speak—it's hard to see how good nurses catch errors or early signs of decompensating, communicate with patients and the health care team, and prevent disastrous outcomes. There are many formers patients walking on this earth who wouldn't be here today if a good nurse hadn't caught subtle signs early on. These good nurses encourage an entire team caring for separate patients to work together and care about each other's patients just as much as their own. They influence unit culture profoundly. When processes change, good grey nurses don't complain to the group, brush it off, or refuse to adapt. They handle changes with grace. They ask good questions about new processes, suggest edits, and change the way they practice because it has been proven to be safer. They do not hold on to old methods with white knuckles because "that's the way we've always done it."

Being a good nurse truly isn't measured in letters after your name, certifications, professional affiliations, or by climbing the clinical ladder. It's not the amount of money you saved with a research project that identified a cost-savings plan. It's not always being under budget or going a year without a fall. While those things are superb and very important, they are not everything. Good grey nurses not only understand the importance of these things, but also that it takes more than these things to be a successful nurse. You must have a degree of emotional intelligence and truly care about what is best for each patient and make *that* the priority, in addition to all of those other wonderful things. It is truly the blend of the technical and the emotional, the black and the white, that compose a good nurse.

It's a Journey

Having wisdom, grace, and discernment in terrible situations isn't something that everyone carries within them. Not everyone can explain complex medical conditions to an overwhelmed patient. Compassionate care is something we assume all nurses provide, simply because they are nurses. Once you get out there, you'll realize that is not the case.

Becoming a grey nurse is not automatic. It takes going through some rough situations and learning from them. It means gracefully accepting constructive criticism and allowing it to make you better. It means checking your ego at the door. It takes practice, trial and error, and courage. You must be brave enough to be wrong and be okay with yourself if you don't get something right the first, second or third time. You must persist and persevere. You must have enough courage to jump forward, all in, with your priority being to become better every day.

If you do not have the courage to admit mistakes, you will become the most dangerous nurse on the unit. It is essential to release that desire to do things perfectly at every turn if you want to become a successful nurse. There is a lot of trial and error in this journey, and if you beat yourself up every time you make a mistake, answer a question wrong, or do something inefficiently, you will become your own worst enemy. You will leave yourself bruised and bleeding, wondering what nursing did to you, when it was you that was doing the beating.

Becoming a grey nurse is messy. It requires you to tap into areas of your own emotions that are challenging and frustrating. It takes a degree of emotional intelligence to know the most comforting or challenging thing to say, or to know when to be silent. It takes discernment to know how to calm an over-whelmed and scared mother enough to let you take care of her son, or when to encourage, motivate, and challenge a patient to push through an obstacle, rather than continuing to avoid it. Not saying the best thing to someone in crisis or not getting the reaction you thought you would allows you to learn from the situation so you can be better in the future.

Keep in mind, going through some of this may bring up some of your own struggles. It's hard to walk through a patient's worst nightmare and not connect it to your own experience. It will take time to be comfortable going all the way there with patients. You'll know which situations you want to jump all into and ones you must hang back from because of your own emotional needs, in order to safely care for yourself and other patients.

You will get there. It takes time, learning from mistakes, and really appreci-ating successes, but you will get there if you put your heart and soul into it.

Before you know it, you'll be able to reexplain the worst news a husband is ever going to hear because it didn't quite make sense when the doctor said it fifteen minutes ago. And how to comfort and reassure him when you see it click in his mind that his wife is forever gone.

You'll know when to just sit and listen to a man tell his entire life story after he just learned that he's essentially dying slowly. You'll know how to make him feel important, valued, and cared for. You'll know that is now your priority, not charting the assessment you just did on your last patient or seeing if your coworker needs to go to lunch.

Physicians will trust your instinct.

You'll know how to make coworkers who hate each other work together.

You'll know how to quickly grab control of a room full of frantic people when things start going downhill. You will know how to convey urgency, not terror. You will somehow make others in the room feel safe when someone's death is literally a breath away. You'll have calm confidence because, even if the worst of the worst happens, you can handle it. You will become an amazing problem-solver, be able to critically think elbow-to-elbow with the physicians, and be able to tell when a family member doesn't need another explanation of the pathophysiology of the cancer that's killing their dad, gently redirect conversation, and support that loved one.

Your presence will put both coworkers and patients at ease. At first, you'll be focused on getting things done textbook correctly (the black side); it'll take a few situations of emotional discourse to really palpate the white side of nursing. Once you really feel it, you will know it's there, like a hematoma or subcutaneous emphysema. You can read about these situations, but once you feel it yourself, you have a better understanding. When you feel what it's like to stand with someone who just found out their spouse passed away, you begin to understand just how to act in those situations. You will start to put the pieces together and understand how to best support patients in those tough emotional situations and not just get through them. You'll then be able to transform from that brand-new nurse focused on the black side to a nurse who understands the white side as well. Finally, your blend of nursing grey will be so glorious that before you know it, you'll be your unit's own Gandalf the Grey, BSN RN.

Everyone will be happy to see you're working on the same day as they are. You'll be able to handle any situation that may come your way with ease, confidence, and grace. You'll go from a seemingly average nurse to the nurse patients will never forget because you were there for the tough times. You'll make Gandalf so proud that he'll come to your one hundred and eleventh birthday and set off the best fireworks display this side of the Shire.

One of the beautiful things about nursing is that some nurses are better at some things and some are better at others. A nursing unit is quite the team. I am somewhat the emotional supporter on my team. I have some colleagues who are great at technical stuff (IV insertions, Foley insertions, placing sutures, etc.), some who are great at having crucial conversations (calling a doctor back when they're not being responsive to a patient's issue, pushing back on staffing when we need another nurse), and some who are great educators (can explain complicated medical conditions to people with little education). It is really lovely to see a well-functioning unit work together, utilizing each other's strengths to best serve our patients.

Everyone comes into their own Gandalfness differently, with their own expertise in the mix. I've accepted that I won't be the best technical-skills nurse, but I really come through for patients and loved ones with emotional needs.

I love when I'm working with my technical nurse who has a calm demeanor, my crucial-conversation nurse who calls anyone at the drop of a hat if we need something, my nurse who is basically an educator because she knows so much, and my motivated and proactive CNA. We're like the dream team. How safe would you feel if you knew a team of Gandalfs were manning the unit that your mom was on when she had a massive stroke? No unit feels safer than ours on those days. No matter how crazy it gets, our patients are safe and expertly cared for. It is a beautiful thing. Each of us has had our own journey to become our version of Gandalf the Grey, RN. I know they're all good nurses and I respect and care for them like they're my family—my own Fellowship of the Rings.

Chapter 2

Surviving Nursing School

I had absolutely no clinical experience prior to nursing school. Other than providing first aid to the kids who fell on the pool deck during my summers as a lifeguard (despite telling them walk 12 seconds), I had no experience being responsible for the care of another.

Therefore, my first clinical experience was utterly terrifying. I started getting nervous the week before. I tried to prepare as much as possible, but nothing could prepare me for what lay ahead.

Nursing school provides you with a lot of firsts. I'd like to share with you two of my firsts—my first bed change and my very first assigned task in clinical.

My first bed change

You know how people say nothing can prepare you for children? Well, nothing can prepare you for changing a bedbound 300-pound patient who cannot move and is covered in feces and urine in a small, unventilated nursing home room. Nothing.

Before I could begin real nursing clinicals, I had to become a certified nursing assistant (CNA). This meant completing nursing home clinicals, the down and dirty work. Feeding, bathing, and cleaning patients were the priorities, things with which I had absolutely no experience.

My patient for the day was a larger woman with advanced dementia. She could not speak or follow commands. She had lived in the nursing home for the past ten years. Staff informed me that family rarely visited her. Basically, her life consisted of lying in bed and being turned and changed every few hours by the nursing staff. She was fed three meals a day by a nursing assistant. That was it. That was her life, which was quite the reality shock for my first day of clinicals. While I had heard of this before, I had not actually seen it for myself. Reading about it in school is quite different from looking at a living, breathing person in front of you and knowing that is their life.

Nevertheless, she was my patient for the day and I was going to take fantastic care of her—or so I thought. As I came in to meet her for the first time, I smelled a smell I will never forget.

It was the very first time I had ever smelled feces mixed with urine that had sat for a while. It truly made my eyes water. I left the room because I was in shock and had no idea what to do. Well, I did not what I needed to do, I had no idea how to actually go about doing it.

"How do you even move someone this large in this small of a bed to... you know... really clean all of the -gulp- areas that need to be cleaned?" I thought. I went to find my clinical instructor for what I thought was necessary guidance but was actually, at least to her and other nurses in the facility, just common sense. I seriously had no idea how this was going to work, and I certainly didn't know how people did this multiple times for her and many other bedridden patients all over the world day in and day out.

"I think she has gone to the bathroom," I quietly and sheepishly told my clinical instructor.

"Welp, better go get some supplies and someone to help you clean her up!" she said with a smirk, like she waited every year for the reality of nursing to smack the new students in the face. I honestly don't blame her; I bet it was pretty entertaining to see me looking like a confused puppy.

I grabbed what I thought I needed and found the first poor soul who emerged into the hallway. Thankfully, it was one of the nicest people in my nursing class. She was happy to help me and I was ever so thankful.

We were both first-timers. This was the first time for me changing anyone in any capacity (no one in my family had children younger than me, so I'd never even changed a baby diaper at this point), and the first time for her changing an adult.

We looked at her like she was a puzzle, unsure of which piece to pick up first, as we tried to remember our simulation training.

Spoiler alert: Simulation training is to real nursing care as Mario Kart is to driving. It merely provides a peek into the environment; it is not at all like actually doing it yourself.

My classmate held the patient up on her side with all of her might in that tiny, poorly ventilated nursing home room to reveal the extent of the task that lay before me.

It was more than I could handle.

After I tried to hold in a few gags while my classmate looked away so she didn't see it herself, I reluctantly began cleaning.

My eyes started to water as the smell of stool mixed with urine filled the room and our souls. I tried not to breathe at all, which clearly doesn't work for very long. I tried to breathe inhale short, tiny breaths through my mouth. **Nope.** Dry heaves. Try something else. Shallow breathing through my nose? **Nope.** More dry heaves. I'll try breathing through my mouth again. **Nope.** I'm going to throw up. ABORT, ABORT!

I panicked because I didn't know how to breathe and not vomit on this poor woman. I clearly had not figured how to do the "shallow nurse breathing" trick many of us learn on the job to enable us to get through such situations with a straight face.

I was trapped.

I profusely apologized to my classmate, who had started dripping sweat, and ran to the hallway for a taste of some sweet, sweet fresh air.

Nursing home air never smelled so good.

I took one last deep breath and ducked back in. We fumbled and struggled our way to get that woman squeaky clean. Now, I've had some proud moments in my life, but that bed change was truly one of my shining moments. However, the reality began to set in that this was not something that happened infrequently. This was a normal, everyday aspect of nursing. The blood that had returned to my face had suddenly drained again, returning my face to a cool, pale white. I was beginning to get quite comfortable with being utterly terrified.

Afterwards, I found my clinical instructor and had a breakdown moment. "I can't do this! I almost threw up doing the simplest thing a nurse can do!" I was almost in tears.

"You'll get used to it; it'll get better," my nursing instructor replied. I don't know if that was a deterrent or comfort, but somehow I felt better.

The man, the student nurse, and the condom catheter

As nursing school continued, things escalated to the more complex. Twice a week for eight hours, eight of my classmates and I met at a local hospital on its medical-surgical unit for our first actual nursing clinical experience. On our first day, we were all very nervous. None of us knew what to expect.

Thankfully our clinical instructor was kind, hilarious, and a phenomenal teacher. We truly hit the jackpot. Once we were acclimated to the unit, she asked for a volunteer to complete a task. Determined to be an awesome student, I immediately volunteered.

"Great!" she excitedly said in front of the entire group. "We're going to go put a condom catheter on a male patient down the hall!"

"Um. Okay," I nervously replied. "I've never done that before. What do I need to do?" I was terrified and confused. I honestly couldn't even remember what a catheter was at that point.

As she showed us the condom catheter in her hand, I started to realize it was a little more straightforward than I had anticipated. "Well, have you ever put on a condom?" she loudly asked in front of all eight of my classmates, whom I had just met the week prior.

With redness engulfing my face from embarrassment, I awkwardly replied, "No, I haven't."

I wanted to blurt out, "Hey guys, I'm one of those 'wait 'til you're married' type of girls," but thought day one of clinicals with people I met one week ago was just a little too soon. So, I just endured the stares and confused looks until my blushing face calmed back down to that terrified pale white I was becoming accustomed to.

I'm not sure if the extremely personal question even fazed her. After all, she was a nurse.

We walked into the room and there sat a frustrated sixty-something-year-old man. He'd had a stroke the day before and was having trouble doing anything he used to because he had lost function on the left side of his body. The frustration he felt with this situation was taken out on the staff at every turn. No one could win with him.

Something he was used to doing completely independently up until twenty-four hours ago was use the bathroom. Now he could not control it and kept urinating all over the bed. His skin had become raw and the staff had to go through bed change after bed change. A condom catheter was the solution to his problem, but he wasn't too thrilled about it. They'd gone through about four of them because he just kept pulling them off because they didn't "fit right."

Well, guess who was about to reapply his fifth condom catheter? Yes, ladies and gentlemen, little old me on day one of clinicals.

My clinical instructor, one other student, and I headed in. My instructor explained what was about to happen, and the patient just grumbled in reply. He knew the drill. He knew he needed it, he just wasn't happy about it.

I put my gloves on, pulled the sheet back, and lifted his gown.

"You're going to feel cool down there," said my clinical instructor to the patient, who didn't seem to notice. She instructed me to coat him with skin prep (something that makes the catheter stick), and I rolled the condom catheter on.

Now, I don't mean to brag, but that catheter stayed on all day, a feat not achieved by any nurse previously. Nursing school is all about little victories and that man and his condom catheter were mine for the day.

I took what I could get.

Organization

Nursing school is all-consuming. With frequent exams over hundreds of pages of material, multiple weekly clinicals, math exams, board reviews, and extensive prerequisite requirements, you barely have time to ruin the recipes you find on Pinterest anymore. (Quite the tragedy, I know.)

I was a typical B student: Not the top of my class, not the best test-taker, the kind of student who woke up eight minutes before class every day. Not a slacker but not trying to fight to the death for every single point either. After going through school and a certification exam, I learned that one of the biggest keys to successfully getting through nursing school is appropriate organization and planning.

Once you get all your syllabi (and recover from the subsequent myocardial infarction), get a calendar and write out all due dates for the entire semester for each class. Write this on a calendar you will look at every single day. This may be one on your phone, your wall, or in a planner. Get a big picture of what is expected of you for the entire semester at once. This is really important because you may have a week or two here and there in which multiple larger assignments or exams are due on the same day. Gone are the days when you could look at what's due for the upcoming week or next few days, study a little bit, and be good to go. There is just way too much information to not only read, but understand, analyze, and apply.

Look at all of these due dates and begin to plan. Plan when you will write your papers. Plan when you will study. Give yourself ample time to do these things, with a little wiggle room in case something isn't making sense and you need to go in for your professor's office hours or touch base with classmates.

This will have a few benefits. First, by not only planning when you'll study but also planning the specific topics you will study during this time, you'll become more efficient. You won't spend the first twenty minutes just trying to pull your sources together to study. You'll know exactly what to study so you can sit down and start immediately. Second, because you know you've allotted the time you need to study, you will be able to relax more because you know you've planned out when to do what. You can look at your schedule and see where you can fit in a workout, a mental health day, lunch with a friend, or whatever you desire.

I started nursing school with the mentality "When in doubt, study," which left me studying all the time. This was an inefficient use of time because I was overworking myself and inefficient in my studying. Had I planned appropriately, I would have had more effective study sessions and seen when I had time to relax more, which would have enabled me to focus better when I actually was studying.

As far as organizing your materials for coursework, use whatever system works for you. I would color-code topics, use a hanging file folder, and flag frequently used texts for quick navigation. The desktop of my computer was organized with a folder for each class, each of which had subfolders for each section to be able to quickly find things. It is important to organize both your electronic and paper worlds, otherwise you waste a lot of time just looking for things. It may not save you a lot of time initially, but this can add up to saving you a few hours a week.

You also want to be able to go through old coursework to find things as you begin really studying for the NCLEX. It was really helpful to be able to pull out my folder from my previous class about a specific topic when I got an NCLEX practice question incorrect. As you're finishing courses and moving through the program, make sure you leave those materials in an organized fashion. This includes disposing of papers you know you won't need (trimming the fat, as people say) like rosters, notes you've transcribed somewhere else, explanations of assignments that have already been completed, and so forth.

As Scar from *The Lion King* would say, "Be prepared."

Studying

Before nursing school, I would focus on getting through reading assignments before exams. However, in nursing school reading the material won't be enough. You are bombarded with deep concept after deep concept, like perfusion, oxygenation, ventilation, pH balance, and so forth. Therefore, you really have to stick to your plan about what to study when. Your studying plan must include time to read the important pages and also time to process and understand that information.

These blocks of time to study should be short. Don't make the typical mistake of setting aside six hours the night before an exam. It's really tough to concentrate and retain information for that long at one time. People retain information best in twenty- to thirty-minute increments. Close your tabs, turn your phone on silent, turn off the TV, and focus intently for those twenty- to thirty-minute blocks of time, then give yourself a ten-minute break to check Instagram, grab a snack or some fresh coffee, or do some yoga stretches. Then, back to it! Doing that for two to three hours will be much more effective than staring at a book half-paying attention for six hours.

Additionally, figure out how *you* learn best. Some people like to hear things over and over again, while others like to read, highlight, and type, while others like to read and explain or watch a video. Not everyone learns the same so one method isn't better than another. I used to get frustrated when someone else could record a lecture, listen to it a few times, and ace an exam. While that was great for them, it wasn't how I absorbed information best.

Relationships

Nursing school is quite demanding. It can put strain on relationships with friends and family and it can be tough to navigate new relationships with classmates, professors, and clinical instructors as well as figure out how to talk to patients.

When your friends and family are not the ones physically going through school, it can be tough for them to really understand how demanding it is. Communication is essential with loved ones, those that you live with, or with those upon whom you depend significantly (a spouse, parents, and so forth). It can be especially beneficial to let them know ahead of time what is expected of you. Maybe show them your calendar so they can see everything laid out. Having those tough, "Hey, I really want to be present for you as much as possible but while I'm in nursing school, I won't be able to do as many things" conversations is a lot easier before you're frustrated with each other than in the midst of a heated moment.

Navigating all of these new nursing school relationships can also be challenging. Clear communication is essential with everyone. If you do not understand an assignment or concept, go to your professor's office hours and talk it out. When I initially went into college, I felt this barrier between my professors and myself. I was intimidated to talk to them when I didn't understand something. I looked at class and clinicals as a performance where I had to show them all I knew with as little help as possible. However, this is not how learning works. I needed to get over my hang-up about impressing authority figures and be honest about the things I didn't know. Years later, after talking with many educators and hearing their perspectives, approaching it this way is essential to growth. Educators want people to communicate to them when they don't understand something. This is how they know where to elaborate more or how to change their style to enhance understanding.

I want to really encourage you to view class, clinicals, and office hours not as a time to show what you know or perform and avoid correction, but as a time to take in new information and learn. Embrace correction and teaching. Be honest when something doesn't make sense. Educators, clinical instructors, nurses you're shadowing, and patients don't always know if you've fully understood what they've said. "So what I hear you saying is _____. Is that what you mean?" is a really helpful way to make sure you're hearing what they're trying to say. Honestly, my husband and I say that to one another when we're discussing something but don't seem to be on the same page.

Additionally, you're going to be in class with the same people for quite some time. You may also find yourself in clinical groups, group projects, and online discussions. You will get to know one another very well. It can be tough to be in such close proximity to people for such an extended amount of time and not get frustrated with one another. I get it. I've been there. However, it is important to get into the habit of not talking about each other and not judging one another while you're in school. This truly requires skill. It takes some practice to see someone behave in ways that frustrate or annoy you and not go vent to a friend who knows them and would understand.

Harnessing the ability to not engage in this behavior takes practice and time. It may even be something you have to unlearn from younger years. However, it could not be more important. If you are regularly commiserating with classmates about other classmates, this will translate into your work life upon graduation. When you're new to a nursing unit, it is natural to want to connect with other people as fast as possible so you feel welcome and comfortable. Some people like to bond with others over people they don't like or understand. It's easy to quietly express frustration to the person sitting next to you in lecture. This can quickly build a tiny bond, even when you've not really had a chance to get to know the person yet. A smirk, a laugh, or an eye roll between one another opens the door for an inside joke. Therefore you begin relating to one another, and conversation naturally begins to flow.

This is an incredibly dangerous culture to cultivate in nursing. This eventually translates to the "nurses eating their young" issue and unhealthy work environments, which ultimately affect nurse satisfaction and patient care.

If this is something you find yourself doing, start disengaging with this in nursing school, so you don't fall into it when you get your first job. It is much easier to change this in school, rather than when you've been on a nursing unit for five years and developed a reputation among your colleagues. Also, if you are commiserating with colleagues about others who frustrate or annoy you, this easily crosses over to your patients. This mentality can prevent you from being able to see past their decisions, their disease processes, and their culture and render you incapable of providing them the nonjudgmental care they deserve. You'll be frustrated with the patient who attempted suicide, annoyed with the noncompliant diabetic, and roll your eyes whenever you get a patient who wants to do a prayer ritual you've never seen before or asks about using alternative therapies.

I don't think anyone starts out in this career with the goal of becoming a judgmental nurse. This is something that slowly happens over time. It begins the first day of orientation, when you're trying to bond with the people near you over a common interest. Many times that common interest is the annoying guy up front who keeps asking questions, the girl behind you who smacks her gum and smells, or the know-it-all. It can be funny and innocent at the beginning but if that's how you initiate relationships, people begin to expect that behavior of you. People will look to you for your response in various situations like a new policy, when a new employee starts, when someone does something questionable, or when a patient acts funny. People will look at your response and then formulate their response accordingly.

This produces a mentality on the unit that discourages honesty. People will be too scared to admit when they don't know something because they're scared of judgment. Because they want to just fit into the status quo, people don't speak up. They end up pretending they know everything when they really have knowledge gaps and educational needs. Ultimately, patients suffer.

A safe nursing culture is based on honesty and professional accountability. Staff must have the permission to be honest and imperfect and to make mistakes. Otherwise, people spend so much time pretending and saving face that they don't even know what they don't know.

It is imperative that when people come to you with questions and uncertainty that you make these teaching moments and not times to bond with others by making fun of the questions asked. Responding with grace, even if you think it is something this person should know, is the foundation of professional accountability. We will not hold each other accountable, receive constructive criticism, and change our practice if we are too worried about being judged and talked about in a negative light.

This isn't something that comes easily, especially if you've been doing it for the last twenty years. This change can be challenging, but it is possible. It requires accountability from your loved ones and cohorts as you commit to improvement. Let people know you're trying not to do this and ask your friends to call you out when they see it.

This honesty between friends is essential to personal and professional growth. Give your loved ones permission to bring things to your attention. Respond with gratitude, reflect on what happened, and apologize when you mess up. Being humble about mistakes and honest about your weaknesses speaks much louder than trying to be the seemingly perfect nurse.

The bottom line: Be honest when you don't know something, be graceful when someone asks you a question, and treat your colleagues with the same nonjudgmental attitude that you provide your patients.

Care Plans

Care plans were always very challenging for me in nursing school. For those of you who have not yet had the frustrating challenging of writing one, they are the essence of the nursing process, expressed through nursing diagnoses, interventions, rationales, and outcomes. They guide your nursing care for the shift. Now, years into my career, I can quickly create one in my head, but in nursing school, it was one of the most challenging assignments.

After gaining some perspective about care plans, I've come to a few conclusions.

First, they are necessary. Some nurses out there are very vocal about how we don't actually use these in the real nurse world. The reality is that we do use them each and every shift, we just don't realize it. In the emergency department (ED), nurses complete care plans at lightning speed. When we turn our patients every two hours, prevent them from falling, have a plan to address their pain, facilitate a bowel movement, or have a conversation with them about their anxiety, we are implementing a care plan.

Second, I want to reassure you that it is normal for these to be challenging in nursing school. It is really hard to understand the normal nursing diagnoses for various patient populations if you're not used to seeing them yet. If you don't know the typical nursing diagnoses, it's hard to know the expected rationales, interventions, and outcomes, and how to evaluate it all. It should be something that's difficult in school because you just haven't seen a lot of patients yet.

Give yourself plenty of time to complete care plans. Trying to crank one out the night before it's due may not work well. Capitalize on your professor's office hours if you do not understand it. I used to get really focused on the wording of the care plan. While this is important, it is not the only thing that matters. The information contained in NANDA-I, Nursing Intervention Classification (NIC), and Nursing Outcomes Classification (NOC) is based upon the standardized terminology used to write these care plans.

Essentially, NANDA-I, NIC, and NOC are lists of standardized terms that you must use in your care plans so that a nurse creating a care plan in North Dakota is using the same language as another nurse in Florida. It makes sense to have this standardization, but it does make it a bit challenging for those of us learning it for the first time. It is kind of like learning another language, when you know what you want to say but you just don't know the right way to say it. Because of this, it is really easy to get inundated with the language, rather than focusing on thinking like a nurse. The goal is for you to get report on a patient, meet them, come up with some practical goals and a plan to help them progress during your shift, implement it, and then evaluate it.

Therefore, when you're going through clinicals, think practically about what things you want your patient to do today and how you want them to progress. Do you want them to have better pain control? Do you want them to have a bowel movement? Do you want them to walk three times and sit in the chair for all three meals? Do you want to be able to discontinue their restraints? Did they verbalize any specific concerns or knowledge deficits? If you focus your mentality on how you want them to progress and on addressing any verbalized issues, rather than the specific wording, it will make coming up with a care plan much more fluid.

Figure out what you want to say in plain language, then translate it into the NANDA-I, NIC, and NOC terminology. Eventually, you'll get much more used to the standard terms and you'll start thinking in this terminology, making this process much quicker and smoother.

Nursing School Clinicals

Clinicals were another challenging aspect of nursing school for me. As I mentioned before, I had very little hospital experience before nursing school. Being exposed to the clinical environment for the first time was like Aladdin showing me a whole new world. Except there were fewer talking monkeys, flying carpets, and genies, and more catheter insertions, bodily fluids, and documentation. Below are my tips for getting the most out of the clinical experience.

Befriend the nursing assistants

When you're starting out and learning the basics, an experienced certified nursing assistant (CNA)—occasionally referred to as a patient care technician (PCT)—can be your saving grace. They know the unit and the patient population very well. They know how to give an amazing bed bath. They feel very comfortable in the clinical environment. They know the ins and outs of the beds, supplies, and staff. The nurses you will shadow and work with will focus on things like meds, care plans, diagnoses and so forth, but the CNAs can show you how to give quality basic nursing care, which you absolutely must know. Remember, just because you are working toward a nursing license doesn't mean you are above giving a bed bath, washing someone's hair, or taking them to the bathroom. The sooner you're comfortable with basic nursing care, the better—and the CNAs can expedite this process significantly.

Take initiative

Don't just stand up against the wall in the hall waiting to be told what to do next. Find things to do. Tidy up the patient's room, talk to the physician who's rounding, see if you can help a CNA with a bed bath, ask to observe procedures. Speaking as someone who has worked with nursing students in the past, it is very frustrating to have a student with you who completes a task and sits down and waits to be told what to do next. Take initiative to get the most out of your clinical experience. No one will take initiative for you. Remember, nursing is a team sport. We care for all of the patients on our unit. It is not one nurse caring for their patient load in their own little silo in the corner. We answer each other's call lights, give meds for one another, get labs, and so forth. Therefore, if another patient needs something, jump in and see how you can help. Also, make sure the nurses you're working with know you want to help. Saying something like "I'm new to this whole clinical thing and want to be as helpful as possible, so if there's anything I can help you with or anything that needs to be done, please tell me. I may not realize some of the things that need to be done yet" can really open the line of communication with someone new you're working with.

Always have a quick snack nearby just in case

It is inevitable that a nursing student passes out during clinicals. I get it. I've been there. You feel really worked up and nervous, so you don't eat breakfast and at the first sight of an IV insertion, blood draw, or pus-filled wound, you hit the deck. This is why it is so important to have quick food to eat on the go, a granola bar, nuts, fruit, or whatever works for you. Clinicals are also very busy and you may not get time to eat for hours, so it's nice to be able to grab the granola bar in your bag and quickly eat that whenever needed.

Ask questions

Clinical instructors and bedside nurses don't always realize when you don't understand something. When things are really fast-paced, it can be hard to communicate when something isn't clicking. Make sure you're asking questions or for further clarification. Most people are in a mode to teach and welcome questions. If they aren't, still ask them or find someone who will explain it to you. Remember, this is your learning experience and occasionally you'll need to advocate for yourself to get the answers you need to understand something. Please do not get into the habit of not verbalizing when you don't know something. Be honest, dig in, and truly understand what's going on. Please do not view clinicals as a performance where you always have to know the answer. This is a learning environment where you're being exposed to things for the first time. It is okay to not know.

Be respectful of the staff

Typically you'll complete your clinicals on various nursing units. I've seen a lot of behavior in the past that really frustrated me, from the nursing student who asked the CNA to "help" her with a bed bath as she just sat back and let the CNA do all of the work, to the student nurse who couldn't stop talking about how he "would never work in a unit like this," to the senior BSN student who condescendingly corrected the ADN-prepared nurse (who had fifteen years of experience) at every possible turn. I could go on and on. But really, just make sure you're being courteous and respectful of the people who have chosen to work on that unit. Everyone has different experiences, education, and qualities they bring to the table. Everyone has value. Therefore, just because something is not valuable to you (like experience on a specific kind of unit) doesn't mean it's not valuable to someone. Please, treat everyone with respect.

Be prepared

Have everything you need with you. Check, double check, and triple check before you walk out the door. Have the correct uniform (a pair of backup scrubs in the car doesn't hurt), a snack, pens, a small notebook, stethoscope, and anything else your school requires. Having a small notebook that fits in your scrub pockets can be really helpful because not all instructors will allow you to use your phone. Even if they do allow you to use your phone, they most likely won't allow you to use it in front of patients and visitors. However, whenever I overheard something I wanted to write down—a lab value, memory device, explanation of something that finally clicked—I was always in a patient's room. Having a notebook on hand enables you to take notes in the moment wherever you may be. You always think you'll remember something, then another call light goes off and it's forever gone from your brain.

In addition to notes for assignments, labs, or just little helpful tidbits the nurses would provide me during clinicals, I'd also write down talking points. If I really liked how a nurse explained something to a patient, how they were firm but kind when someone was rude, or how they advocated to a physician on behalf of a patient, I'd quickly write that down so I would remember. Those talking points were so valuable because they helped me communicate things I felt but didn't have the words to say.

Communicate with instructors

The clinical environment can be pretty intimidating, especially if you've never had clinical experience before. Therefore, if you suffer from anxiety or any other health issue that you think might affect your performance, let your instructor know. It is a lot easier to explain that you have anxiety beforehand, than in the moment when they ask you a question in front of everyone and your face gets hot, your heart starts pounding, and you get cold sweats. Let them know that you may need a little more time to answer questions and that this doesn't mean you don't know the answers, just that you're already working to keep your anxiety at bay so it's a bit more challenging to recall that information.

Also, as I said before, make sure you communicate when you don't know something. Many instructors begin to explain things and then move on when there are no questions. Maybe you didn't have a question at that time, but later, when you've had time to process the information, it doesn't really make sense anymore. Follow back up and obtain clarification. This is your education—get the most out of it!

Patients are just people

In nursing courses, you learn so much about patients with specific problems and issues. You really focus on doing the right things for various issues. It makes the patient seem so different from us, so textbook, so sterile. But remember, at the end of the day, they are just people. Talk to them like you would talk to anyone else, with respect, kindness, and empathy. You will learn so much about the textbook stuff from the patients themselves. Ask the patient who's been diabetic for twenty years what he knows about diabetes. Ask the heart failure patient what heart failure really feels like and what her biggest challenges are. Ask the patient with severe depression what he thinks has helped in the past. And after you ask these questions, sit back and listen. Don't listen merely to provide a response; listen to understand.

Prioritizing Your Mental and Physical Health

Nursing school is quite demanding and can take a toll on both your physical and mental well-being if you're not being proactive about it. Here are some practical tips to keep yourself balanced during nursing school.

Make time to engage in nonnursing activities

If you're all nursing all the time and only hang out with people who only talk about nursing, you're going to go insane. And your loved ones will get so sick of you talking about nursing that they'll go insane. Make some time to spend with people who are not in your nursing classes. Give yourself time away from the hectic life that is nursing school and de-stress. If you've managed your time appropriately, you won't have to stress about assignments while relaxing. This can look however it needs to for you. Some people de-stress doing strenuous activities, some want to curl up in bed with a good Netflix series to binge, some want to get a massage. Think about what you, not everyone else, would enjoy most and take some time to do it. Advocate for yourself!

Eat well and exercise

I know this tip is pretty predictable, but I promise it is worth it. Eat as healthy as you can while still allowing a few indulgences. If your sustenance is Doritos and Easy Mac and you're staying awake off the fumes of a Red Bull, it'll catch up with you in the forms of constant exhaustion, constipation, and more. Eating healthy not only helps you feel better, it helps your immune system deal with sickness better. Getting sick in nursing school can be pretty stressful because there can be a lot of assignments or clinicals to make up, which is a literal and figurative headache. Take care of yourself by eating healthy foods and getting good rest routinely so that if you are exposed to a cold or flu virus, your body has a better chance at fighting it off.

Also, sitting in class all day, running around clinicals, and studying all night is pretty monotonous for your body. You don't have to do some Ironman workout, but make sure you're getting to the gym or somewhere you can do some good stretches to relieve tension. Lifting weights and cardiovascular activity are also wonderful. The stronger and healthier you are, the easier those twelve-hour shifts will be.

Make time for this. Make your health a priority. Allow time to make a healthy and delicious dinner. Allow time for adequate rest. Run to the gym for a quick workout. Time management and efficiency are key during and after nursing school. A good rule of thumb is to care for yourself the way that you're going to care for your soon-to-be patients.

Have boundaries with your classmates

It's really easy after an exam to try to see what everyone else received. From my own experience, try not to care about how others are doing at every turn. It'll only falsely inflate your ego, or if you're like me, make you feel bad about yourself because you didn't do as well. If you're truly not doing well, go chat with the professor on what you can do differently, not the girl next to you who gets 90 and above on every test and acts like it's no big deal. That'll just make you more frustrated and defeated every time you sit down to study. It can be helpful to see how others answered some questions here and there, but if you're waiting after each exam to see how you stack up, it can become pretty defeating, especially if you're someone who struggles with perfectionism.

Try not to engage in talking about each other when someone shows up late (again), or keeps asking ridiculous questions, or is still mad about a point they missed three weeks ago. That stuff can seem like a big deal in school, but honestly, it's not. Focus on what you need to do when you're there, and don't care about what other people are or are not doing. It truly does not matter. You'll be annoyed at yourself three years later when you think about how much of your time and energy was spent talking about, entertaining, and perpetuating issues that didn't matter. Also, engaging in this behavior is dangerous. It takes the focus off what really matters—becoming a nurse. This is a tough habit to unlearn, but as I said before, it is essential not to engage.

Stay focused on the goal of becoming a registered nurse

There were many times in school when I almost forgot the whole purpose of what I was doing, and it was apparent others had done the same. I think the most evident display of this was when students would spend exorbitant amounts of time arguing with a professor over an exam question. On rare occasions it was worth a bit of respectful dialogue back and forth so we all could learn. However, that was not usually the case. Since I've become a nurse author and blogger, I have received many emails asking, "How do I deal with the frustrating classmate who keeps wasting the entire class's time over a question here or there?" I get why you would want to know the correct answer and work through your thought process. However, you have to ask if this is a valuable conversation for the entire class to take part in or if this discussion would be better conducted outside of class. Honestly, if you are mere points from passing and therefore hypervigilant about every single question, something else is going on. Conversely, if you're getting great grades on exams, it's not a great idea to waste everyone's time in class fighting about something that doesn't really make a difference anyway. The stress that I saw a few points create for certain individuals during school was shocking. You will not get them all right. You will miss points. You will misread a question, mark the wrong answer, or think something was a priority when it wasn't. There will always be a question or two out of left field that no one knows—just accept that it will happen.

Focus on passing and understanding, not on being the best. When you're at the bedside, no one cares what your GPA was. I've never had anyone, outside of two interviews right out of school, ask me that question. Your GPA is important for graduation and getting into graduate school, if that is a goal of yours. Realistically, you should find the balance between not caring at all and being fixated on every single point. Remember that the goal is truly learning how to be an effective and safe nurse. Points are easy to focus on because they are so straightforward, but this is a part of that black part of nursing that I mentioned before, which is only half of it. Put your heart and soul into understanding the information as a whole, passing nursing school and the NCLEX, and becoming a safe and caring nurse. If all you care about is a 4.0, you're doing it for the wrong reasons.

NCLEX Quick Tips

After you are done with your classes and clinicals, walk across the stage, and go through your pinning ceremony, you still have to pass boards. Yes, you have your degree, but it doesn't mean much without being licensed.

It's pretty overwhelming when years of grueling schoolwork culminate into one single terrifying exam. There's no way to completely take the stress out of this ridiculous process, but I think if you approach it with intention, you can reduce the stress significantly. Don't listen to those people who are fabulous test-takers who say prep courses are a waste of money and just bought a $20 book, studied for a night, took it hungover, and passed. They're the exception, not the rule.

I'll tell you a little bit about my postgraduation timeline. I graduated in May and took a full week off after graduation and didn't look at one textbook or think about nursing at all. 'Twas glorious. A short mental break is desperately needed after nursing school. For your sanity, please take some time off.

After one of the best weeks of my life, I took a review course. When my review course began, I put all of my nursing books from school away and focused on the book that was provided. I did what they told me during the course and followed their plan.

I didn't cross-reference things from various books, I didn't buy three additional NCLEX study guides, I didn't cram, and I didn't try to read as much as possible. I encourage you to focus on a few key study materials in addition to a question bank. It's too much information to reference all of your texts from school. Pick a few that are really comprehensive, make sure you understand key topics, and just start answering practice questions regularly.

I answered twenty-five to fifty questions daily for four weeks until I sat for boards. I took one day off per week with no questions or studying (again, sanity preservation). I do not recommend waiting months to sit for boards. The longer you wait, the more you forget. Just get the test over and done.

I took my test three hours away from where I lived in the afternoon during the second week of June. I got great sleep the night before, had my husband drive me so I could relax on the way, and also had him take me out to lunch right before.

I was done in an hour and fifteen minutes and passed with seventy-five questions.

Reminder: I'm not a 4.0 student and not a great test-taker.

Most people walk out feeling like they failed. You'll feel like that even if you graduated summa cum laude and are a great test-taker. You just spent years studying your butt off for every single point, all while getting used to an 80 percent needed to pass. However, the NCLEX is structured very differently than nursing school exams.

I know nurses who timed-out after the six allotted hours and passed. I know those who got all 265 questions and passed in three hours. I know quite a few who passed in 75–120 questions. I know one who passed with 75 questions in 20 minutes.

Pick a study course and stick to it, take days off, test as soon as you're ready, and relax the day before.

If you don't pass the first time, figure out what you need to do the second time around. The world is not over if you don't pass the first time. I know multiple amazing nurses who did not pass their first time. This test does not define your career. I've never had any patient or family member ask me how many times I took my boards. I've also never had a job application ask for that information.

Whether you failed it once or you're going to take it for the first time, now is the time to be disciplined. You must create a plan, focus, and stick to it. There are no excuses, no shortcuts, and no cramming.

Licensure Basics

So you've graduated nursing school, been pinned, taken and passed boards— now what? You still have to physically obtain your license. This process looks different from state to state. I went to nursing school in Iowa, tested in Indiana, and planned on practicing in Illinois. I just assumed this process was something that was part of nursing school. It is not. During your last semester of nursing school, I highly recommend looking up the processes for obtaining your license in your specific state. Each state has a state board of nursing with a website that typically spells out the process required. Make sure you understand what is expected of you and allow time to ask instructors or the board if you have questions.

Essentially, you must apply to your respective state board of nursing (BON) as well as register with the company that administers the NCLEX (currently that is Pearson Vue). You will go to your BON website and apply for licensure by examination and follow their steps. (These steps typically include paying a fee, a background check, and submitting fingerprints and official transcripts.) Concurrently, you'll get registered with Pearson Vue and pay an additional fee. Your BON will determine if you are eligible to sit for boards.

Once the BON deems you eligible, they will send you something called an Authorization to Test (commonly referred to as an ATT). You will utilize this ATT to schedule your test date with Pearson Vue. Please know, ATTs expire, so it would be beneficial to wait until you're ready to test (I do highly recommend testing as soon as you're ready and not putting it off) to apply for one. I also encourage you to familiarize yourself with the BON website in the state in which you'd like to apply prior to graduation so you know what's expected of you, and so that you can plan accordingly and avoid any major headaches.

Coming Around Full Circle

You won't put together the picture you're painting of what it means to be a nurse until you're a few years into your career. You get bits and pieces in school, trying to make sense of it all as you plug along with assignments, clinicals, and many firsts. Your first bed change, your first IV start, your first Foley insertion on a morbidly obese, confused, and combative female patient, your first code, your first death, and the first time a patient at death's door comes back to the unit months later completely healthy to thank you for caring for them during the worst time in their life.

Once you start to walk through these experiences, your picture of nursing will become clearer. You'll be able to understand things on a deeper level. Your critical thinking skills will develop and become more comprehensive. You'll master the basics and therefore won't have to stress about them anymore.

Things that seemed impossible at the beginning will suddenly seem not only possible, but easy. Things that previously took an hour will take at most three minutes. Things that you thought would make you vomit earlier eventually won't affect you. And not only that, but you will be able to go to lunch minutes later and enjoy your meal just the same.

Nursing presents so many challenges, but you have no idea what you're capable of conquering. So when you're in school and think there's no way this can get any easier, hold on to the hope that it will. Before, I was terrified to turn and clean that nursing home patient—I almost threw up. Now I clock-in with confidence, knowing I can handle most situations that will come my way and who to call for the situations in which I am clueless.

Those first few experiences molded me into who I am as nurse. The poopy bed change and the condom catheter were just the beginning of my crazy nursing journey. Oddly enough, I am thankful for those experiences, and thankful and amazed that God has graced me with the desire and the joy to continue.

Chapter 3

Getting a Job

Getting a job in the nursing profession isn't as straightforward as one may think. The expectation that new nurses will be able to walk across the stage and onto the unit of their dreams is unrealistic. While there is a general nursing shortage, there is also a high turnover rate associated with employing new nurses, which is very expensive for hospitals. Therefore, whenever a hospital decides to hire a new graduate, it is a very calculated decision.

There's a lot of planning that goes into finding employment that begins way before you walk across the stage. For this reason it's important to begin searching for your first job *before* the end of your last semester in your program.

Hopefully you have been building connections and relationships (networking) with clinical instructors, nurses, and physicians in the various nursing units in which you had clinicals. Think about whom you would like to ask to write a letter of reference or recommendation for you. (We will talk about this a little bit more later.) In the beginning of the year, typically around January or February, new graduate nurse residency programs start accepting applications from prospective employees.

But what exactly *is* a new graduate residency program?

New graduate residency programs are somewhat new in the field of nursing. It is a structured program for new nurses to progress through during their first year in the profession. They are designed to provide support during the transition from graduate nurse to bedside nurse. I personally went through one in 2010 in Illinois and was very thankful for that experience. That first year is extremely challenging, and it's wonderful to have the support of other new graduates and specific faculty members as you walk through that journey.

I highly recommend applying for a new graduate residency prior to graduation. Why before graduation? These positions open up months before your final semester ends. For example, if you are on track to graduate in May, applications usually become available in January. These typically require quite a few things, so it's definitely not something you can do last-minute. You may have to write an essay, collect letters of recommendation, or even submit a video interview. Regardless of the amount of work, applying for a position in a nurse residence is well worth it.

Depending upon the facility, the program may be structured differently. In my program, we met once a week for four hours and discussed a new topic during each meeting. The educators always checked in with everyone to see how we were doing. Honestly, just sitting around with a bunch of other people who were at the same place in their careers as me was incredibly comforting. Even if we only had the opportunity to touch base with one another, it would have been more than worth it. I have met people who have gone through a new graduate residency program that was an entire year in length. Instead of meeting once weekly, they met once a month. Regardless of how the program is set up, they are great. The best way to find out if the hospital you're interested in has a new graduate residency program is to go to their website. They may have a page specifically for new graduate residency programs or even a page of their employment section specifically for nurses. However, there's typically a specific job posting for a new graduate residency. Once you find the appropriate posting, you will apply for this position specifically. This job posting most likely will not ask for your license number, as they realize you are applying while still finishing nursing school. Applying for nonresidency positions will be somewhat challenging because they typically require a license number, and you will not have one yet.

You do not have to work at a facility with a new graduate residency program to be successful your first year, but I still recommend beginning your job search months before your final semester ends. Most people land jobs because of relationships and networking, so it's important to make a good impression on those that you meet in your clinical environment. If you know you want to work in a hospital where you are currently doing your clinicals, ask around about job availability and what the hospital is looking for *before* your graduation.

Preparation for Job-Hunting: Things to Do Beforehand to Set Yourself Apart and Give Yourself an Edge

Build relationships. As I said before, make sure you're building relationships and rapport with people as you get closer to graduation. It is really helpful to have respected names on your application as references who can speak about your relationship with them in some capacity.

Be thorough. As you're completing your applications make sure you have everything that's needed for them. Be on the ball. This is definitely *not* a time to slack. Typically, there are a lot of applicants vying for a very small number of vacancies in new graduate residency programs. This is especially true for slots in highly coveted units. I cannot emphasize enough the importance of researching these positions as early as December (assuming you're gradu-ating in May) so that you have time to get everything together. I recommend looking at the hospital or facility's mission statement, vision, and values. It is very important that you be knowledgeable of these in preparation for any interviews that you may have. I went so far as to write these down on a notepad I had in a leather binder that I brought to my interview. It's not necessarily realistic for you to memorize the mission statement, vision, and values of each facility you apply to, but it is a good idea to write these things down. It shows that you put in a little bit of time and effort.

Research yourself online. Prospective employers *will* look online and research applicants. Take a look at all of your social media accounts. Survey everything. What kind of picture are you painting of yourself? Do you like what you see? There is no perfect profile nor is there any specific way that you can appear on social media that will magically land you the job. However, there are ways you can appear on social media that can severely damage your chances of getting hired. The manner in which you discuss your profession, coworkers, prior or current employers, work conditions, and so forth can be a career *maker* or a career *killer*. Take a look at your profile pictures and imagine what someone may think when they see them. And yes, this includes screening all of those vacation pictures from Panama City that you posted on your Facebook page. Remember: As a medical professional, you are held to a higher standard of conduct than most other members of society.

Consider a bachelor's degree. To comply with the 2010 Institute of Medicine report *The Future of Nursing*, 80 percent of the nursing workforce should have bachelor's degrees by the year 2020 (IOM 2011). There is currently a move by many hospitals to employ nurses who have graduated with a bachelor's degree. If you do have your bachelor's, that's wonderful. If you do not, be prepared when you apply to be asked if and when you plan on obtaining your bachelor's. If you're able to articulate that you are already in a bridge program or are looking at them, with a goal of graduating in two years that may give you an edge. Keep this in mind.

Gain experience. Something prospective employers really like to see on resumes is experience within *their* facility. This could be in a completely different role, maybe as a medical unit secretary, a volunteer, a phlebotomist, or a pharmacy technician. If you already have a job at or have in the past worked at that particular facility, that gives you a bit of an edge. It could also be very beneficial if you had letters of recommendation or references from people who still work in that facility to advocate for you.

Create a solid resume. The first impression you make on an employer is through your application and resume. It's really important that there are no errors on these. I know it sounds cliché, but you don't get a second chance at making a good first impression.

When you're creating your resume, make sure you have other people review it for you—make that multiple other people, preferably four to six. Be sure to include relevant work history, but do not include every place you have ever worked in your entire life. Furthermore, if you are in nursing school and do not have any experience outside of clinicals, that's okay. It is not necessary to list every single clinical experience on your resume. Employers assume that if you have graduated from nursing school you have a certain amount of experience. What *is* helpful to include on your resume is clinical experience related to the specific unit to which you are applying.

It is also important that your resume be concise. For example, if you worked as a certified nursing assistant in a nursing home, it isn't necessary to explain that role in an essay underneath its listing. A single straight-to-the-point sentence is sufficient. You don't need to explain that you provided exceptional baths and therapeutic communication, fed residents, and so forth in multiple sentences. I have included some resources relevant to resumes in the resources section.

Prepare for interviews. Interviews can be quite intimidating, especially if you have to complete peer interviews. Let's go over a few things that are important regardless of your interview panel.

First, it's important to look good when you are interviewing. You don't need to go buy an expensive new suit, but you do need to look like you care. If you feel the need to get a new blouse or update your shoes, do it. I cannot stress enough the importance of looking well-groomed. Again, you don't have to go spend $500 at a local spa before coming in, but you do need to look like you've showered, that your hair is clean, your facial hair is tamed, your clothes are clean, and so forth. People can tell when you make the effort to look good for something important. The person(s) interviewing you can tell when you have put in the effort to look professional.

Also, keep in mind that during this time, it's important to make a good impression on everyone. Don't only worry about the person(s) actually interviewing you. Be considerate of the person who runs the front desk of the HR department, the person taking your picture, or the person showing you where to go for the interview. I know people who will ask the receptionist what they thought of someone who came in for an interview. With this tidbit of information fresh on your mind, be careful how you conduct yourself in person or during cell phone conversations (especially when you think no one is listening) while in the waiting room prior to your interview. Treat everybody with respect and make a good impression on all.

You also want to keep in mind that your first impression was made on your application and resume. Your second impression was made, not during the interview, but when you were contacted to set up an interview. If it is difficult for the human resources department or the nursing unit to get in touch with you to schedule an interview, or if all of the dates they offer you are not doable for you, you aren't making a great impression. They realize that you have a life and things going on, that you can't drop everything to schedule an interview, and that it may be incredibly difficult to find times that fit your schedule. But they also have many others applying for the same spot. Keep that in mind.

In addition to looking great and making a good impression when you walk in, your demeanor is also really important. It's important to be confident but not cocky. While you don't want to highlight everything you've done wrong, you do want to be humble. I call this being humble and hungry: I'm humble in that I know I have a lot to learn, but I'm hungry to learn these things.

Arrive early. If you are unfamiliar with where to go, it might be beneficial to do a dry run the day or two before. Show up a few minutes (more than fifteen minutes is overkill) early for your interview. Introduce yourself and shake hands.

I personally like to carry extra copies of my resume along. I have been to one or two interviews in which my resume was misplaced. Had I not been able to hand them a new copy, they would have had to look at a wall while interviewing me. It also looks really great if you're able to hand them a resume on actual resume paper.

In my leather portfolio, I keep a notepad. A few days prior to the interview, I research and take notes on this notepad so that I can refer to them during. Things I include are the mission statement, vision, and values of the particular facility I'm interviewing with, any possible notes for patient scenarios, as well as questions I have for them. I want to make sure I have all of this information at hand.

This next bit may sound silly, and you may feel like you don't have to do this, but I highly recommend that you make up possible interview questions and practice answering them. More likely than not, you will be asked questions about patient scenarios. After going through nursing school, you would think you'd remember all of the scenarios and be able to recall them easily when asked. However, mid-interview, when you're really nervous and trying to look the best you can, it's hard to recall all of those experiences quickly. Therefore, I encourage you to practice some questions at home before the interview. Here are some sample questions:

- Tell me about a time you had to advocate for a patient.
- Tell me about a time you made a mistake. How did you handle it?
- Have you ever had to do service recovery? Tell me about the situation.
- Why do you want be a nurse?
- Why do you want to work at this facility?
- Why do you want to work on this unit, specifically?
- Tell me about three of your greatest strengths.
- Tell me about three of your greatest weaknesses.
- Tell me about a time you had to do something for a patient and you weren't sure how to go about it. How did you handle that?
- What are your long-term and short-term goals?

It may be beneficial for you to take some quick notes on your notepad that correlate with some of the questions.

- **Advocacy:** Lady who fell on hip, called MD four times for different pain meds
- **Service recovery:** Tracked down a meal tray for an hour

- **Experiences:** Assisted with central line placement on forty-year-old intubated pneumonia patient
- **Weaknesses:** Too big picture, slow to catch on, not used to working in a large team environment
- **Strengths:** Adapt quickly to new technology, experience with charting system, not afraid to take initiative or have tough conversations

OK, now I'd like to talk a little bit more about the three strengths and three weaknesses questions. I want to encourage you to have real answers for these questions. Speaking as someone who has conducted new graduate nurse interviews, nothing frustrates me more than when someone gives very cliché answers to these questions. Don't say that you work too hard, you care too much, and sometimes you're too interested in your job like Michael Scott from *The Office*.

I encourage you to sit down and think honestly about the things that you need to improve on and if you can articulate those in a graceful way during an interview. For example, when I applied for a position in a neurosciences intensive care unit (ICU), one of my weaknesses was that I had no idea how to work in critical care. I had a big learning curve ahead of me compared to someone else with more experience. However, I countered this weakness by saying that I was very willing to learn and excited for the opportunity to do so. Another one of my weaknesses is that I am a "big-picture" thinker. I don't get caught up in details, even though sometimes I should. This can be a positive attribute, as I do not get overwhelmed by the little tasks because I am constantly thinking about how they are part of the big-picture goals. However, there are many details that are essential to critical care that sometimes get lost in my big-picture thinking.

Also think about your real strengths. Saying "I'm a hard worker, I care about my patients a lot, and love nursing" doesn't really tell me a lot about you. But if you say something like "I'm really efficient," or "I'm good at reading the emotional climate of the situation," or "I'm very good at picking up new procedures quickly," you will reveal much more about yourself. It shows me that you take these questions seriously and actually put some thought into them. Interviewers notice and appreciate this. Remember: Your goal is to stick out in a sea of applicants. You want to be memorable. You do this by being honest, genuine, and unique.

I once interviewed someone who was very nervous. However, I realized that being interviewed for a job is a very nerve-racking experience, so I tried to make them feel at ease. This person answered questions well, even though they did so nervously. Then I asked a question for which they did not have a prepared answer. This person sat quietly then said, "Let me think on that for one moment. I am not sure if I have an answer to that." So, we sat there for a second or two. It was slightly awkward but not too bad. After a few seconds, they said, "You know what? I don't have an answer." I know this person did not answer the question, but their honesty about not having an answer really spoke to me. So, in my opinion, this person, who was nervous and didn't actually answer every question, had a pretty good interview, and after all the interviews that day, that was the person I wanted working on our unit. This just goes to show you that you don't have to be perfect in interviews, but you do have to be genuine, polite, on time, appropriately dressed, and considerate. All of those things require not talent but effort.

When they ask you to give specific patient scenarios, the interviewer really just want to hear about you and your experiences. I interviewed an individual who, when asked about a scenario, talked about how the previous nurse or another nursing student screwed up. After about four or five questions, I started noticing a pattern: Everything was somebody else's fault. Wow! This person had the hallmarks of a good interview: they spoke well, had their binder and their resume, and were well-dressed, confident, early, and polite. However, I did not like that every answer was about somebody else screwing up. I wanted to hear this person's strengths, things that they did well, and what they took away from the situation. If you have to utilize the faults of others to increase your appeal, there's a problem, and I'm going think twice about having someone like that on my team.

Brainstorm questions for the interviewer. Interviews always conclude with the interviewer asking if you have any questions for them. *Always* have questions for them. I repeat: Always have questions for them.

Remember: You're not just anybody. You're a hot commodity. You're a wonderful employee to have, and this institution would be very lucky to have you. It is a two-way street. You bring something to the table. You may be interviewing at other hospitals and the hospital across the street has better tuition reimbursement or a higher nurse satisfaction rating. If you don't ask, how will you know? Think about what you want in an employer and see if they are willing to provide that.

Sample questions:

- Do you offer tuition reimbursement?
- Are bachelor's-prepared nurses compensated differently?

- Do you encourage specialty certifications? Do you provide any financial assistance for nurses obtaining their specialty certification or bonuses for those who do?
- Do you have a clinical ladder program? How do you encourage professional development for bedside nurses?
- Are there any nurses on the Board of Directors?
- What is the turnover rate of this facility? What is the new graduate turnover rate?
- What is the turnover rate in other units that I'm applying to? How long has the nurse manager been here?
- When did this facility obtain its Magnet designation? When is it up for renewal?
- What percent of nurses at this facility are nationally certified?
- What is the average nurse-to-patient ratio? Has this average changed recently?
- What is the average length of orientation for new graduate nurses?
- Is incivility or bullying a problem on this unit or in this hospital as a whole?
- Is there a shared governance council on the units or facility level?
- Is there anything about my application that concerns you?

The Follow Up

Alright now, stick with me. We are almost to the finish line. I know you might be thinking as soon as you walk out of that interview that your job is done and you just have to wait. Wrong. There is one last thing that you need to do.

You must send a handwritten thank you note.

What? A handwritten thank you note? Is she serious?

I am absolutely serious. Remember, you must set yourself apart. Just imagine: The person interviewing you also interviewed sixty other people that week. Over the next week or so, think about those other interviewees. Those people are also hoping for a second interview. What if, during that week, that little handwritten thank-you note was the deciding factor on who got a second interview?

I recommend doing this for whomever you're interviewing with. I did this for the nurse recruiter and the nurse manager. If the hospital requires multiple rounds of interviews, it doesn't have to be some long, fancy, or elaborate thank-you note. Just a quick little card that sincerely thanks them for their time is all that is necessary.

> ### *Thank You Note Example*
>
> Dear ____,
>
> Thank you so much for taking the time to interview me for the open nursing position on your _____ unit. I enjoyed meeting you and learning about your team. I appreciate your time and consideration. After getting to know you and learning more about the unit I believe I would make an excellent addition. I believe that my _____ make me a perfect candidate. Please feel free to contact me with any additional questions.
>
> Again, thank you for your time and consideration.
>
> All the best,
>
> _____

I hope these tips will help you in your job search. As I write these words in 2017, the market can be somewhat tough for new graduate nurses, depending on your location. Therefore, you must set yourself apart from all of the other applicants. You must be diligent at every step of the way. This will pay off when you are starting your new graduate orientation while others are still frantically searching for jobs after graduation.

Reference

Institute of Medicine. 2011. *The Future of Nursing: Leading Change, Advancing Health*. Washington, DC: The National Academies Press.

Chapter 4

Graduate Nurse Turned Bedside Nurse

The Normal Learning Curve

The learning curve is somewhat steep when you start this phase. You are going from learning about nursing theory, theoretical instances, and very general concepts to engaging with very specific and practical situations. You're getting to know the physicians, the nursing assistants, your colleagues, computer systems, the supply room, what the supplies are called, as well as the different resources and personalities on the unit. There is a lot to learn!

Naturally, when there is so much to learn, you are going to be very task-focused. You are going to be honing in on how to do the little nitty-gritty tasks. You are going to be worried about how to administer blood, how to start IVs with the specific equipment in this unit, how to use the phone system, how to document, how to use the medication dispensing machine, how to draw labs, how to get your patient a tray of food at specific times of the day or night, and so forth. The list goes on and on. However, after a little while you will get a lot faster and better at completing these tasks. The tasks that once intimidated you, that you thought would take hours to complete, will soon become second nature and you will completely them seamlessly.

For example, at the beginning of my bedside career, if I was going through my shift and all of a sudden saw orders to start a Heparin drip with boluses on one patient, had another patient's family member on hold, had a physician making rounds, and had another patient on the call light asking for pain medication, I would be pretty overwhelmed. After some time on the job, I began to feel more confident handling all of these situations quickly and efficiently. You will get there too. Don't get discouraged at the beginning when you're unable to foresee problems, put clinical pieces together to predict a possible outcome, or anticipate needs. It is hard to pull that all together when you're so worried about just completing tasks correctly. It will come.

Typically, by the end of orientation your confidence level will have grown, and you will be able to complete most tasks easily, anticipate situations, and think critically. While you may not be operating at lightning speed, you will be efficient as well as *proficient*. However, you will always have room to grow in the area of critical thinking.

Basic Orientation Structure, Preceptors, and Mentors

The way nursing orientation is structured varies from facility to facility. However, there are a few commonalities that I will go over.

First, orientation will be a specific number of weeks. When I completed my graduate orientation in 2010, I had a twelve-week orientation. I felt that was sufficient. It was neither too long nor too short. I felt very supported by my team and was ready to be on my own by the time I completed the program.

You and another nurse will have to sign off on the various competencies. Competencies are documents that specify various tasks that you must demonstrate your ability to complete safely per the institution's policy. Examples of these competencies include IV insertion, medication administration, central line discontinuation, central line dressing changes, and peritoneal dialysis. The list goes on and on. The competencies that you will be responsible for depend heavily on the unit where you work. Therefore, the competencies for a nurse working in an operating room will be very different from a nurse working in hospice.

You will have a preceptor. This is someone whose job is to insure that you become a safe and efficient caregiver at that facility and on that specific unit. This is a somewhat formal relationship. This person is involved in completing formal evaluations, educating you, correcting you, and so forth. They are your hands-on, at-the-bedside educator. At the beginning, your preceptor will be showing you the lay of the land, so to speak. They will show you how things on that particular unit flow. As orientation progresses, they will be less and less hands-on. If orientation is going well, by the end of it they should basically be sitting at the nurses' station the entire shift checking behind you. At this point, you should be essentially functioning independently.

What your preceptor is not is another person to taking care of patients with you. It's not the two of you tackling an assignment together. Ideally, as you progress, your preceptor will be backing off. Their goal is for you to feel encouraged, empowered and able to take a full patient load by the end of orientation safely and independently. This cannot happen if your preceptor is doing tasks for you. Even if, in the moment, it would be faster for your preceptor to page a doc, grab a set of vitals, or hang some intravenous fluid really quickly, it is essential that they let you manage your time and allow you to figure out how to do it all yourself.

Communication is key. If you need your preceptor to help you a little bit more, explain a few more things, or give you more opportunities, they need to know that. Conversely, if you think that your preceptor needs to back off, is doing too many tasks for you, or is not allowing you to function as independently as possible, thereby inhibiting your growth, they need to know that as well. They may not realize they are doing that. This is why throughout orientation you should be checking in with them and monitoring your progress. Naturally, this relationship can become a little strained. Becoming a nurse is very humbling. Expect to be corrected a lot during this process. It is the preceptor's job to correct you and to ensure that you are completing tasks and procedures safely.

Additionally, you should also have a mentor. A mentor and a preceptor are two different things. Your preceptor cannot be your mentor, and your mentor cannot be your preceptor. They function very differently. If you get along well with your preceptor, that's wonderful. However they still cannot be your mentor. While you and the preceptor should have a very business-like, formal relationship, the relationship with your mentor should be comforting and friendly. Your mentor's priority isn't to get you to become a functional nurse on the unit. Their priority is to make you feel welcome, assist you in acclimating to the culture, and support you emotionally through this trying process.

I recommend meeting with and talking to current nurses on the facility's staff about this process. Open up the lines of communication with your colleagues. It's always nice to have someone else's perspective, especially from someone who's been through it. Walk through different situations with them, describe your thought processes, and get their opinions. But most importantly, get their support. This is important because a lot of the loved ones and family members that you normally go to for support will not understand how tough this is. When you start to describe specific nursing scenarios and personalities, they won't understand as easily as someone that's been through it on that unit.

The Role of the New Graduate on the Nursing Unit

When starting on a nursing unit, there's a natural tendency to want to become one of those go-to nurses right away. Again, this takes time, and the way to achieve this is to have a very successful and intense orientation process. As a new graduate in the unit, your educational needs are the priority. Ideally, you and your preceptor are documenting the kinds of patients that you have taken care of, as well as the kinds of patients and situations to which you need exposure.

When you and your preceptor clock in and look at the patient list for the unit, you both should have established a list of the patients you will be caring for that day. While many nurses like to take care of the same patients on a daily basis—this allows them to become more familiar with that patient's norm and makes them more apt to notice any slight changes in that patient's condition—this may be difficult to do with rotating schedules. There are only so many shifts where you will have the guidance of a preceptor. You need these experiences during this time. Your educational needs alone outweigh those of a nurse simply wanting to have their same patients back.

Furthermore, all of the other nurses on the unit should know that you are the new graduate so that if they are taking care of a patient with something out of the ordinary, they know to pull you in and show you what's going on. The more you are exposed to during this orientation time, the more prepared you will be upon completion. Again, your preparedness for this transition is the priority.

Generally speaking, most preceptors are well aware of the importance of your limited time during orientation and look to maximize it. However, not everyone does that. So what do you do if your preceptor doesn't appear conscious of this fact? As stated previously, it's very important to communicate. Do you need them to back off a little bit? Do you need them to support you a bit more? Do you need them to advocate more during your learning process? Do you need them to communicate this information to coworkers so that you can get the experiences you need while you're in orientation? Clearly identify what you need in a way that is respectfully and appropriately communicated. The best time to communicate this is during routine evaluations between you, your preceptor, and nurse manager, that way you have another person there who can support and facilitate the conversation.

Occasionally you and your preceptor may not be a good match. It happens. Just as you have a particular learning style, educators and preceptors have particular teaching styles. While it is important to try to mold teaching styles to the needs of preceptees, sometimes it becomes necessary to switch and get someone whose style better aligns with your needs. Again, the ultimate goal for all parties involved is for you to become a safe and effective nurse, not to build someone's ego.

The Orientation Process

After orienting nurses, taking multiple precepting courses, and observing many more go through the process, I've noticed a common structure. Let's dive into the various phases of orientation that I have observed as very consistent, regardless of the unit.

Phase 1: Observation, or, the lay of the land

During this phase, you're observing your preceptor take care of a normal patient assignment. You're mindful of your preceptor's expectations, how various staff communicate with the health care team, and how they communicate with their patients and the patients' support systems. You notice where supplies are, as well as what the supplies are called as this can vary from facility to facility. This is typically the shortest part of orientation and may only last a few shifts. By the end of this phase, you should be comfortable jumping in and taking a small patient load.

Phase 2: The training wheels are still on

The second phase of orientation is when you start really getting your hands dirty. Hopefully you've already begun taking a patient or two, or more, depending on the unit that you're working in. You begin taking reports on these patients. You walk through your thought processes, your priorities, and your time management with your preceptor. Be thankful for this and take every opportunity to ask questions and take notes. During this phase, be prepared to make mistakes, to do things inefficiently, and to screw some stuff up. This is all part of your learning process. It's expected. It is also expected that you will learn from your mistakes.

You continue to complete and sign off on competencies. I highly encourage you to keep copies of these for yourself, even though many times a copy goes to your manager. It is important that you have your own documentation as well in case something happens to the original. Even in the digital age, things still manage to get lost. The last thing you want to do is have to redo forty competencies.

As you're learning these new tasks, promote your own independence. Identify the experiences that you need as well as your weaknesses. These exercises are really important and rely on you knowing what experiences you need and your comfort levels with various tasks. For example, if you're nervous about admissions and typically forget all of the things that you need to gather, make overcoming nerves a goal of yours. When you're up for the next admission, ask your preceptor to hang back and observe you, but not help you. See if you can independently remember all of the tasks that you need to do to success-fully admit the patient. Then ask your preceptor how you did.

It is essential that you are honest about your educational needs and not faking perfectionism. Try to fight the natural inclination to save face and look like the smartest and best nurse. That'll only get you so far. It is really important to identify what you don't know so that your preceptor can help fill in the gaps. They will do their best to teach you all you need to know in order to be successful. If, however, you're not communicating with them about what still isn't clear or what you aren't comfortable with, it can be difficult for preceptors to identify your specific needs. This phase of orientation, when the training wheels are still on, is the time to be honest with yourself and attack your shortcomings and deficiencies head on.

Phase 3: Try and fly

As you continue to progress during this process, your preceptor will step back farther and farther, allowing you to operate more independently. Eventually you will be taking report independently on your patients and jumping right in and doing what you know more frequently. Your preceptor should be hanging back and observing what you're doing and only correcting you when neces-sary. You are the primary nurse for your patients. Your preceptor is merely checking and confirming your actions. Remember: you are the nurse caring for your patients, not you and your preceptor. I have seen various well-meaning preceptors attempting to help their orientee by completing tasks for them. Do not allow this, especially this far into orientation. It is essential that you learn to manage your time and responsibilities.

Goal Setting

Throughout this entire orientation process you should be setting SMART goals. These goals should be ones you set with input from your preceptor. These should be a combination of what you need to know to be safe in the unit, identifying your current abilities and level of competence, and what you struggle with.

SMART Goals

Specific:_____

Measurable: _____

Agreed upon: _____

Realistic: _____

Timeframe: _____

Source: Doran, G. T. 1981. "There's a S.M.A.R.T. Way to Write Management's Goals and Objectives." *Management Review*, AMA Forum 70 (11): 35–36.

Some examples of SMART goals include:

Phase 1

- By the end of this week, I will be able to confidently answer the phone at the nurses' station, know how to put people on hold, transfer calls, and field questions.

- By the end of this week, I will be able to log into the medication-dispensing machine, remove medications, return medications, and be able to properly dispose of narcotics.

- By the end of this week, I will be able to settle a new admission, hook them up to the appropriate monitoring, and take and document basic vital signs.

Phase 2

- By the end of next week, I will be able to start an IV and document this appropriately and independently.

- By the end of this week, I will be able to complete a full head-to-toe assessment and document such appropriately in less than thirty minutes.

- By the end of this week, I will be able to participate in interdisciplinary rounds, submit reports on my patients, and field appropriate questions.

Phase 3

- By the end of this week, I will know how to access urgent override medications and administer these appropriately in an urgent or emergency situation.
- By the end of this week, I will be able to take reports independently on all of my patients, complete all of their assessments, and administer their morning medications on time, unless an extenuating circumstance presents itself.
- By the end of this week, I will acknowledge and implement all new orders within one hour of receiving them, unless an extenuating circumstance presents itself.
- By the beginning of my last week of orientation, I will be giving and receiving reports independently, as well as caring for my patient load independently.

Practical considerations

There are other really important practical things to make sure you address during orientation. These include making sure you know how to schedule yourself, how to obtain your schedule, and how to request days off. It's also important to know how to use and check your email, as well as any other form of communication that your facility utilizes. Use your orientation time to familiarize yourself with non–patient care computer systems. Other computer systems include incident reporting, work requests for equipment malfunctions, communicating and paging other members of the health care team, access to your benefits, and other things like that.

During my own orientation, I didn't fully appreciate how important it was to learn the scheduling software. I came in one day during orientation, began working, and finally noticed that everyone was talking about our schedules being due today. I had failed to realize that this was one of my responsibilities. I found myself frantically putting my schedule together. I was already behind and overwhelmed. I never made that mistake again. I made lots of others but never that one.

Learn your time management style. Time management is an important thing to learn in orientation, and you'll probably have a slightly different style than your preceptor. Take note of how your preceptor and your coworkers manage their time and create your own style. It's important to develop something that works for *you*. I will talk more in depth about this subject later.

And finally, pay close attention in your documentation courses at the beginning of orientation. These are incredibly valuable. Documentation is something you can become efficient at and therefore spend less time doing. As you become more proficient, you will become more confident. Your increased confidence will lead to your development of tricks and shortcuts. Exploit these to your best ability.

Read those emails regarding software updates and learn to optimize the computer system. Whatever you learn in orientation may change significantly over the next few years, especially as far as documentation goes. Computer documentation systems used by hospitals, just like phone apps, update with new functions and features. These software updates often have new capabilities that make other processes smoother, faster, and easier. Pay attention when you see these emails in your inbox.

If you're feeling overwhelmed by learning all of these non-bedside tasks, check in with your mentor. It can be helpful to try to get your mind around these things when you're not in middle of a busy nursing shift. Hopefully, you're regularly meeting with a mentor for additional support and guidance, and you can ask them about how to submit your schedule, check your email, or documentation tips.

Walking through the orientation process is quite challenging for a variety of reasons, but if you have an engaging preceptor and the support of a mentor, it can make all the difference.

Chapter 5

Nurses: Coordinators and Leaders of the Team

Nurses are truly the leaders of the health care team. The nurse is at the bedside twenty-four hours a day, seven days a week, and everyone comes to them about the patient to touch base and receive updates. While the physician sees the patient and puts in the appropriate orders, it's up to the nurse to implement them while balancing all of the patient's priorities. To liken this to basketball, the physician is the head coach while the nurse is the point guard. The physician is calling the plays (putting in the orders), but the nurse is the one physically doing it.

While having this responsibility is wonderful, it can be hard to learn to lead when you're new. Being an effective point guard on day one isn't going to happen. It takes practice. Orientation is your time to practice for the game, which starts the first day on your own.

Another added challenge is that the health care team is large. Instead of leading four other people down the hardwood, you could be leading and coordinating over ten. I'd like to outline some major players on the team so you feel more prepared to step into this important position.

When I started out, members of the health care team would come ask me for updates on the patient. But at that point, I really didn't know what information they were looking for specifically. Let people know you're new and ask specifically what information they would typically expect from the nurse.

> **Physical therapist:** "Hey, can I see Mr. Smith in 82?"
>
> **Me:** "Hi, I'm Kati. It's nice to meet you. I'm actually a new nurse and not sure what kind of information you need typically. Can you let me know what you're looking to know specifically about Mr. Smith for an update?"
>
> **Physical therapist:** "Oh yeah, sure. I'm Josh by the way. I just need to know how he's doing getting out of bed, if it's clinically appropriate for me to see him, and if he's been walking twice a day and up to the chair for meals."

People are usually more than happy to help navigate the newbie; you just have to open that line of communication. Otherwise, they may not realize you're a new nurse and that there's a learning curve. This also immediately begins to build rapport, which is a wonderful thing to do right away.

Keep in mind, not all patients will see every single member of health care team. The physician may order various members to be consulted as they are needed or as it is identified by you as a nurse through a screening process. For example, if the patient expresses financial concerns, many facilities have protocols in place in which the nurse can consult a social worker without having to speak with a physician first. This is not universal and varies from facility to facility.

Additionally, after a member of the health care team other than the nurse or the physician (a physical therapist, dietician, chaplain, etc.) sees the patient, they complete an assessment that includes their recommendations and plan. Part of this plan is the frequency with which they will round on the patient, which is usually indicated in their note. I have had patients and family members become very upset with me when the physical therapist (PT) didn't see them every single day. However, when I pulled up the note in their chart, I saw that PT was only ordered to see them three times a week.

It is essential to communicate this frequency to the patient; otherwise, they can feel forgotten, neglected, or like you're not doing your job, which ultimately causes them to trust you less. It's much easier to proactively educate and tell them what to expect than try to backtrack. There are no replays. You must get it right the first time.

Therapy Services

There are different kinds of therapists who see patients in hospital. These include physical therapists, occupational therapists, and speech therapists. Each of their roles is different; however, they are all very important. When any of these individuals are consulted, they will complete an assessment of the patient in order to understand where they are at baseline and then come up with goals and a plan. This is somewhat similar to how nurses assess their patients and come up with their care plans. Let's go ahead and differentiate between these three roles.

Physical therapist

A physical therapist is someone who focuses solely on the reduction of pain and restoration of mobility. For example, the patient who has had a stroke and now has left-sided weakness will need a physical therapist to assess their needs and come up with a plan to get the patient back to as high a level of functioning as possible.

Occupational therapist

An occupational therapist differs from of the physical therapist in that they focus on optimizing the patient capabilities to complete activities of daily living (ADLs). Their focus is on getting patients back to doing the things they need to do to take care of themselves as independently as possible. For example, going back to the patient who had a stroke and now has left-side weakness, the occupational therapist would focus on tasks like feeding themselves, bathing, and toileting.

Speech therapist

A speech therapist is also called a speech language pathologist (SLP). These individuals work with patients who have impaired swallowing for various reasons (like stroke, various surgeries on the throat, trauma, other neurological injuries, and so forth) as well as difficulty speaking. Difficulties with speaking are rather complex issues. The patient can have an issue speaking clearly, understanding what is spoken to them, or verbalizing words. Speech therapists are able to assess the degree of difficulty the patient has with both speaking and understanding the language spoken to them, and come up with a care plan to restore as much function as possible.

Social Work and Case Management

Social workers and case managers are wonderful resources for the bedside nurse. Frequently, case managers are also nurses! These individuals can help with a lot of outside resources to ensure the patient is supported from various perspectives upon discharge. This can include finances, home health, equipment, rehab, or transfer to another facility, like a skilled nursing home. Their roles differ but they work together a lot and complement each other well. Some of their responsibilities may overlap.

The social worker focuses more on social issues or problems the patient may have. I've utilized them when I was worried about abuse or legal issues regarding my patient, or if I was worried that they were not going home to a safe environment.

The case manager works with the entire health care team and the patient to help determine any outside agencies that might be necessary upon discharge. They are concerned with the overall big picture of discharge and the best scenario for this patient. So if a patient suffered a stroke and has profound hemiparesis, the case manager would work closely with therapy services to see if the patient is safe to go home and has the appropriate resources or if a rehab facility would be more appropriate. They would look at the patient's insurance, speak with patients and their support system face-to-face, get signatures, fill out paperwork, set everything up for the patient's loved ones to visit various facilities, and so forth.

Chaplaincy and Spiritual Support

A common misconception about chaplains is that they can only provide spiritual support from a Christian perspective. However, that could not be farther from the truth. Hospital chaplains typically have specialized training in supporting people in crisis, and many are trained counselors. They can help people process emotions, practice reflective listening, and just be another sounding board for the patient or loved ones as they are faced with big decisions.

Additionally, if the patient or support system are of a particular faith, chaplains have the resources available to find the appropriate spiritual leader. I've had patients from a wide variety of faiths and just called down to the chaplaincy office to figure out how to get whomever the patient would prefer at the bedside as soon as possible. It is a wonderful support to the nurse, especially in larger urban areas where there are many different local temples, churches, mosques, and so forth.

It can be helpful to communicate to the patient that the chaplain's focus is not to come to the bedside and talk about their own particular religion; their goal is to simply provide support. They may not want to see the chaplain because they simply don't want to explain the whole painful situation again, which is understandable. However, not wanting to explain the situation shouldn't prevent them from getting support they need. There can also be added value from getting support from someone outside of the situation, someone who isn't a family member, a physician, or the nurse.

Here's an example of a talking point to the patient or family member you believe may need some additional support:

> Would you like to chat with someone and process this information? I know it can be pretty overwhelming and sometimes it's helpful to talk about it with someone outside of the situation. Gloria, our chaplain, is a great sounding board and trained counselor. Would you like me to see if she has some time to come by?

And don't forget that the chaplains are there to support the staff as well. Once, I was taking care of a dying man with children who were about my age. I was barely holding it together and the chaplain was rounding. She spent ample time with the family, and afterward came and checked on me. She said, "Kati, you know I'm here to take care of you too."

That's it. That's all she said.

I took a deep breath and thanked her as my eyes filled with tears. It made all the difference for me. I was trying to hard to just get everything done, but I really needed to just stop and reflect on what was happening so that I could be more present for the family. Her support and acknowledgment of the situation was all I needed to get through the rest of my day and be there with his family when he passed away a few hours later.

The Pharmacy Team

I love pharmacists. I rarely go a shift without speaking to one. They are an invaluable resource for the bedside nurse. Whenever I have questions about IV compatibility, allergies, dosing questions, and honestly anything that has to do with meds that I don't know the answer to, I chat with a pharmacist. Some hospitals even have a pharmacist specifically for the critical care unit, which is wonderful, because there are quite a few high alert medications that are given in the critical care environment that require special expertise.

There are also many pharmacy technicians. They address mixing and obtaining meds, as well as issues with the medication-dispensing machine. I think I was as well acquainted with the pharmacy technicians as I was with the pharmacists. Nurses and the pharmacy team go together like dates and bacon: You wouldn't think they go together, but they so, so do.

Additional Team Members

There are more people who might be seeing a patient than what I've listed above. Additional members of the team potentially include dietitians, respiratory therapists, nursing assistants, medical unit receptionists, safety attendants, child life specialists, and care coordinators within specific service lines like oncology or stroke.

The bottom line is that there are a lot of members of the health care team. You as the nurse are the home base for that patient. All of these members will come see the patient and then go to other patients, while you are with the patient all day. Frequently, when these members of the health care team would like to see the patients, they speak with the nurse first to make sure it is clinically appropriate or a good time. For example, a physical therapist will usually touch base with the nurse before working with the patient (especially in the critical care environment because things change so quickly). They rely on the nurse's clinical judgment to know if it's safe to work with the patient that day.

Working with Physicians and Their Support Staff

Before I go into some very specific details and tips about working with physicians and their support staff, I'd like to define the roles of everyone who may be working on this team because it is not as straightforward as it may seem. I went into nursing assuming that a doctor was a doctor and that was that; however, there are admitting physicians, attending physicians, consulting physicians, interns, residents, medical students, and advanced practice providers like nurse practitioners (NPs) and physician assistants (PAs).

> *Pro Nurse Tip:* When I started, NPs and PAs called themselves "midlevel providers"; however, this is no longer an acceptable term, as it implies they are above the nurse and below the physician. Terminology differs depending on the facility, but the most consistent acceptable term I've come across is "advanced practice provider."

I also had the opportunity to interview a physician about his experience with and opinion on communicating and working with new nurses. I have included some of his thoughts and input in this section. His name is Rustin Meister, MD, and he is a pediatric resident who currently works at Vanderbilt Children's Hospital in Nashville, Tennessee.

Admitting physician. The admitting physician is the person who decides to admit the patient to the hospital. Frequently the admitting physician and the attending physician (defined below) are the same person. However, there are a few instances in which these are two different physicians.

Physicians within their own group will take turns admitting patients when they are consulted. For example, let's say there are six cardiologists at one hospital in the same practice. A patient comes into the ED and the ED physician decides that this patient needs to be admitted and consults cardiology. Whichever cardiology physician is doing consults that day will come take a look at the patient and the chart and decide whether or not they will admit them. If this happens during the day, routinely the person who admits the patient is the attending. However, sometimes this can change if there's another physician in that group who subspecializes in the specific problem the patient is having (like a neurosurgeon subspecializing in brain tumor removal or a cardiothoracic surgeon subspecializing in valve repair). This may also change if a large number of patients come in a short amount of time. If this is the case, they may change the attending physician just to spread the work so one physician doesn't all of a sudden have ten new patients while another only has a few.

It's important to differentiate between these two physicians because someone may ask who admitted the patient originally, and just because one physician admitted the patient doesn't necessarily mean they are taking over as attending. Therefore, you cannot look at who was listed as the admitting physician and assume that they are also the attending.

Attending physician. The attending physician is in charge; they ultimately call all of the shots. They assess the patient, come up with a plan, and consult physicians from other service lines as needed, all while maintaining the role of the primary physician for the patient. (Examples of service lines include neurology, nephrology, general surgery, cardiology, and so forth.)

Typically, this is a hospitalist or internal medicine physician. However, if a patient was admitted for a particular surgery, that surgeon will most likely be the attending. For example, if they get admitted for a brain tumor that needs to be removed, the neurosurgeon may be the attending. If the patient is admitted and needs a coronary artery bypass graft, the cardiovascular surgeon may be the attending.

"The attending could also be a medical subspecialist," Dr. Meister adds. "Not all hospitals are divided this way, but in some cases subspecialty services have their own admitting services; then, the attending is a specialist."

Consulting physician. As the attending physician deems necessary, they will consult physicians from other service lines. So, if the patient was admitted for a brain tumor by a neurosurgeon but has a bunch of comorbidities, the attending physician most likely will consult the internal medicine team to manage those issues so they can focus on the management of the brain tumor. The physician from internal medicine is the consulting physician.

Dr. Meister also notes, "A consulting physician rarely calls the shots. They offer recommendations that the primary team usually goes along with, but they don't have to." He cautions new nurses that they "may see a consulting physician in their patient's room telling them what they want to do, but the primary team may not think it's necessary." This is why it is essential to touch base with the attending physician or primary team because it is ultimately their decision. Some hospitals do not even permit consulting physicians to enter orders, therefore requiring attending physicians to enter all orders. From a nursing perspective, I appreciate that because sometimes it can be a headache to get orders entered due to physicians not wanting to step on toes.

Medical student. A medical student is someone who is in a graduate-level medical program; they are not a licensed physician. Frequently medical students are observing in the hospital environment. I personally have only encountered a handful of medical students, and every time I did, they were always observing.

Dr. Meister was a medical student not terribly long ago and notes that "medical students [do] very little what [he calls] the manual labor of medicine (what nurses do) or the practical part of medicine (what residents do). Medical students have the most to learn from nurses, but sadly none of that is important to them until they become residents, because it won't be on their test."

Intern. An intern has completed a medical degree and is in their first year of training or residency. They can also be called first-year residents as well. They are physicians, but they still are under supervision and typically not licensed.

When asked about his experience as an intern, Dr. Meister mentions that he "never learned more in [his] life than [his] intern year." He admits that "you go into the job knowing some of the right answers, but not knowing how to actually 'do' anything." (Sound familiar nurses?)

He shared with me a little bit about his first day: "My first day on an inpatient rotation I had to put in orders on different NICU babies. You know how many orders I put in before that? Zero. Utterly terrifying."

Dr. Meister urges nurses, both new and experienced to "be kind to interns. They better be kind to you! They have way more to learn from a nurse than vice versa."

Resident. Residents are people who graduated from medical school, completed their internship, and are essentially undergoing on-the-job training. You may find yourself working with a team of residents who are taking care of your patient. This team can include a first-year, second-year, or third-year resident (the chief resident). As you can tell, it can get kind of confusing. Therefore, it's really important to know the chain of command in your specific facility and which resident to call for what needs. Dr. Meister adds that "second-years can be the primary resident taking care of your patient or they could be supervising multiple interns, depending on the service."

 Please note: If you do not work at a teaching hospital, you most likely will not run into medical students, interns, or residents.

Fellow. A fellow is a physician who has completed a residency in a general field of medicine like pediatrics, internal medicine, general surgery, or family medicine. One they receive that training and want to become a subspecialist within their chosen field, they do a fellowship and become a fellow. Examples of this include a pediatric resident who wants to become a pediatric cardiologist would complete a pediatric cardiology fellowship, or an internal medicine resident who wants to become an oncologist would complete a hematology-oncology fellowship.

Physician's assistant (PA), nurse practitioner (NP): This is a person who has completed a master's-level program. Their scopes of practice are somewhat similar to one another. There are some differences; however, I'm not going to go into depth on those. Another term for them is "advanced practice provider." Many physicians with whom I have worked employed PAs and NPs. The most common structure I've run across is that each physician would have a specific advanced practice provider assigned to them. This advanced practice provider would round on patients, admit and discharge patients, place orders, and work autonomously. For most situations, I would frequently page the PA or the NP first. Most of the time, they were able to address my need. However, there were times where they recommended I called the physician directly because it wasn't a question they were able to address themselves.

While this may sound like a lot of people to keep track of, once you get used to the structure and how everything flows, it's much easier to manage. I enjoy working with residents because they're also in a learning mode. It's nice to become acquainted with a hospital system and patient care with others who are learning themselves. I also love working with advanced practice providers. They are a wonderful resource for the bedside nurse because many were nurses in the past and therefore are great at anticipating nurses' needs. This is also a great career option for nurses as well, if you are looking into graduate school.

Let's go into an example of a patient being admitted to the hospital through the ED and which physicians would care for them based on their circumstances (see box on next page).

So, Who Ya Gonna Call?

No, not Ghostbusters... but I'm not going to lie, I would really like to call them when my patient needs something.

When you're trying to figure out who the heck to call, you need to think critically for a moment. If you have a question about an existing order, check to see which physician ordered it originally.

If this is a new issue, there are multiple physicians consulted, and you're not sure, think about which service is the most appropriate to address the problem. If it's a question about insulin and a surgeon is the attending but medicine is consulted, you should call the medicine physician or the advanced practice provider. If medicine is the attending but you have a question about orders for surgery in the morning, you should call the surgeon's NP or PA. This isn't always cut and dry. I've had times where I had a blood pressure

Example of Admitting a Patient through the ED

A patient is admitted with severe leg pain. After performing appropriate diagnostics in the emergency room, it is determined that the patient will need to have a femoral-popliteal bypass. The cardiovascular surgeon admits the patient and plans to operate tomorrow. However, this patient takes many medications for his uncontrolled hypertension and he is in acute renal failure. The cardiovascular surgeon (the attending doctor) decides to consult the hospitalist (the consulting physician) for medical management. After surgery, the patient's condition declines. The patient needs dialysis, has been noted to flip in and out of uncontrolled atrial fibrillation, and, despite starting Cardizem, continues to have an uncontrolled heart rate. After speaking with the cardiovascular surgeon (attending), the hospitalist decides to consult nephrology (consulting) to manage his renal failure and cardiology (consulting) to manage his cardiac issues.

Attending: cardiovascular surgery

Consulting: hospitalist, nephrology, cardiology

When a patient begins to have complex medical issues after a surgery, occasionally the surgeon will ask the medical physician to take over as the attending physician.

issue with my stroke patient with a significant cardiac history. So I called the cardiologist about it and they told me to call the neurologist. Then I called the neurologist, who turned around and told me to call the cardiologist back. It can get kind of confusing, and I've had a few times where I've had to push back when a physician isn't answering my question, even though they're the most appropriate person to do so.

Dr. Meister's tip for this, if you're calling about a new problem, is to see which resident has been writing notes daily, as this is most likely the person who you would need to contact about an order.

How Their Schedules Work

Typically the medical team does not work in twelve-hour shifts like the nursing staff. I'm going to explain a routine schedule that most physicians on the inpatient setting follow, but please know there are exceptions to this structure.

The attending physician typically works 0800–1700, Monday through Friday. Basically they work normal business hours. During the off hours, the on-call doctor is available. So physicians and their advanced practice providers will round once a day on your patient. The time at which they round is completely up to them and is frequently unpredictable. Surgeons typically have surgeries throughout the day and will try to round on the patients already on the unit before, in between, and after surgery. Other physicians have to work around their scheduled procedures and whatnot. They have a long list of patients, and have to round on (see) all of them. They'll take a look at the chart, talk to the patient, and make any necessary changes.

"In a teaching hospital," Dr. Meister adds, "the resident will often pre-round on their patient, coming to see them early in the morning before rounds so they can present them." You may want to maximize this time to touch base with them about concerns or needs before actual rounds begin later in the day.

Patients and loved ones always want to know when the physician will be around. I have worked with many physicians, and not one of them had a schedule by which I could tell a patient exactly when the physician would be making rounds. There are just way too many variables to provide an accurate prediction.

I tell families when they can roughly expect to see physicians; however, I always say that, if an emergency or something of that nature has occurred, they may not be by during their typical time. It's really important to communicate this to families because if you tell them that the physician will be by around 1000, the family will make sure to be at the bedside at that time. If the physician is not there at 1000, the family may start getting upset and frustrated. Prevent this entire situation by never saying a specific time, rather a general timeframe and always use the caveat, "But if an emergency occurs, this can delay them without notification."

During nonbusiness hours, the on-call physician must be available for any needs. Physicians take turns being on-call. This enables them to rotate call schedules, so that they are able to go home and get some sleep, ensuring they're not essentially working twenty-four hours a day. It's important as a new nurse to know the call schedule, how to access it, and how to speak to the on-call staff. Keep in mind: If you have to call the on-call physician during these off-hours, they may not be very familiar with your patient. If they are not familiar, it is important to give them a brief explanation the patient. Dr. Meister mentions that "patience with physician's cross-covering is important, but if they use that as an excuse to not be helpful to you as a nurse, that's a problem." I'll talk more about tips for calling physicians later.

You may need to page the on-call physician through their office, which would include calling the office's on-call service and providing some basic information. They will put a page out for you.

I like to save my nonurgent needs for when the physician rounds on my patient. However, if it starts to get close to 1700 and the physician has not rounded yet, I will go ahead and call. I do this because after 1700 (or whatever time it is at your facility) if you need a physician, you must speak with the on-call physician. If you call the on-call physician for a routine need that should have been addressed by the rounding physician, they can get frustrated and may instruct you to wait and ask tomorrow when your physician is available. This makes sense because the patient's primary physician should be making these routine decisions, not the physician on-call.

Something I learned pretty quickly is that physicians do not like to step on one another's toes. Some will make some minor decisions and approve some orders for you during the off-hours, but unless it's a pressing issue, most will have you wait until the next day. Please do not take it personally if the on-call physician won't fulfill your request.

Now, I don't want you to think that you'll be stranded between the hours of 1700–0800. If the patient needs something that cannot wait, that should be addressed by whoever is on-call. However, if you're calling at 2100 because the patient wants to restart all of their home meds and ask questions about their prognosis, that's something that's much more appropriate for the primary physician to address the next day. (Dr. Meister emphatically agreed with this point!)

I have had only a few instances in which physicians were so concerned with crossing another physician's boundaries that important decisions were delayed. I ended up having to step in and advocate that someone make a decision so I knew how to proceed; however, that has only happened a few times.

Rounding with Physicians and the Medical Team

Try to round with the team as they see your patients. It's not always possible, but when you're able to do this, it is very beneficial. If you round with the doctors, you can consolidate your needs and concerns all at once while they are with the patient. I like to do this while the physician is completely focused on my patient at their bedside. This way the medical team and I are able to have one fluid conversation about all needs at once. There's no fractured communication of seven pages throughout a shift about nonurgent needs; it's one conversation.

"We value nursing input so much during this time. It's so helpful to hear the plan, raise concerns, and move on. It avoids so many needless pages and phone calls back and forth later," Dr. Meister adds.

Every morning when I get report, I make a list of the things I need to clarify with the physician. I don't immediately page when I find out that I have a nonurgent need. Many things, if not most, can wait until the physician is rounding. Calling every single time you have a nonurgent need is not only an inefficient use of your time, it's also inconsiderate of the time of others. Now, I'm not saying never page the doctors. When you need them, page them. However, if you have multiple nonurgent needs that will not change the immediate care of the patient, or you just need to clarify something, make everyone's life easier and just wait for them to round.

However, keep an eye on the time. If I notice it's 1600 and I've been waiting all day to touch base with this particular physician, I'll go ahead and page them. I want to make sure they'll see the patient before they go off for the night. If they won't be by, then I get all of my questions and needs addressed on the phone at that time.

Calling the Medical Team

One of the tasks I was most unprepared for and the most terrified about was paging physicians. In nursing school, doctors don't want to talk to nursing students. They want to talk to the nurse, get the information they need, and move on. Therefore, few new nurses have ever paged a physician before. I actually completed an informal poll on Twitter recently with some unsettling, but not-so-shocking results.

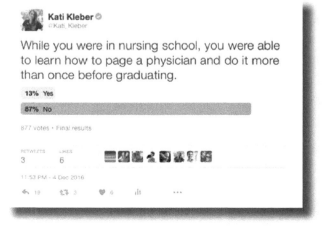

Many responded to me with stories about how scared they were the first time and how they messed it up because they got so nervous that they actually forgot their question when the physician finally called back.

The first time I paged a resident I was absolutely terrified. I didn't even know how to technically page somebody. At our hospital, we would input the ten-digit pager number, wait for the beeps, and then input the number to call back. The first time I didn't put in the pager number right, then, when it was time to input the number to call back, I realized that I didn't even know our unit number yet. So the physician got a page with no call-back number. Then I paged them again and mistyped the call-back number. However, the third time was the charm. I did successfully page them; however, they were not very happy with me. I was so nervous about the multiple incorrect pages that I embarrassingly stumbled through my original question and was just completely mortified.

For those of you who are equally as terrified as I was, I came up with some helpful tips on how to approach this daunting task.

Be prepared. Have a fresh set of vitals, know the patient's allergies, have the labs pulled up, anticipate questions, and be in a quiet area because half the time you can barely hear them because it seems like they are always whispering. It's like you're calling them in the middle of mass or something. If possible, know what order you want. For example, if they've had an increase in premature ventricular contractions (PVCs) and have had a lot of urinary output, anticipate that they may want to check labs. If they're hypotensive with no fluids running and minimal oral intake, anticipate a fluid bolus. Try to know what you want before you call. If you're not sure what they would potentially order, just run it by a coworker quickly. If the patient had their Foley catheter removed eight hours ago and they still have not voided, it would be helpful to know what you would routinely do in that instance.

Make sure you are always critically thinking and not getting too comfortable. If you're on top of your critical thinking game, you can avoid unnecessary pages and therefore significant lags in time management. Dr. Meister says the following about pages from nurses: "I love when nurses know their patients. I love the anticipation too. I feel like it's easy for a nurse to get comfortable and not apply their own knowledge and expertise to a patient because 'the doctor is going to do what they want anyway.' When nurses stop critically thinking, they send bad or unnecessary pages. You are educated and you are valued, you have to act like it and not get lazy."

Don't immediately apologize for calling them. Yes, it not fun that you had to bother them, but it is their job and you're just doing yours. It's all business.

Don't get nervous and just say the patient's name and ask your question. You could be talking to an on-call doctor who may not be familiar with your patient, or they may need a name and a few key pieces of information to jog their memory on this patient. If you're not sure, first ask if they are familiar with your patient. If they're not, give them a brief summary of the patient's main problems. Physicians see a long list of patients and may need a little reminder of what Mr. Brown came in with six days ago.

Let's go through an example of what to say and what not to say when paging a physician.

> **Don't say:** "Hi, Dr. Jones. I am calling you to see if I can straight cath bed 42."
>
> **Rather say:** "Hi Dr. Jones, this is Sarah from 9E. I am taking care of Peter Smith in bed 42. Are you familiar with him?"
>
> "What's he here for again?" Dr. Jones asks.
>
> "Mr. Smith is post-op day three after a femur repair from an MVA. His Foley catheter was discontinued approximately eight hours ago, and he has yet to void. I bladder scanned him, and he has over 500 mL of urine in his bladder. May I straight cath him?"

Don't refer to your patient as their room number. For some reason, nurses refer to patients as their room number (probably because of multiple admissions, discharges, and transfers during one shift). Typically, inpatient physicians see their patients during their entire admission and follow them from room to room; therefore, they always refer to them by their name. So if you call and say, "Hi Dr. Patel, I'm calling about the patient in room 872." They almost always say, "And who would that be?" This also isn't a good habit for nurses to get into, anyway. Try to refer to your patient by their name, not their room number, throughout the shift. Seriously guys, no room numbers. When asked about this topic, Dr. Meister said "Yes, so much yes! Please stop saying room numbers, they mean nothing!"

If it's a recurring problem, ask when they want to be notified again. If you're calling because your patient has had a three second pause with their heart rate in the forties and the on-call physician tells you he doesn't care, ask when he wants to be notified and have an order to reflect that. There are many different policies and protocols that require nurses to notify physicians; however, if it's something that continues to happen, just ask when they want to be notified again so you don't have to unnecessarily bother them or stop what you're doing. They're typically thankful for your consideration when you ask this question. This is also important to carry through from shift to shift, so the subsequent nurses are not continuing to notify the medical team unnecessarily. Be sure to include this information when you give report. And as always, make sure that you're following your policies and procedures appropriately. Frequently patients have multiple nursing orders telling you when to notify physicians during specific scenarios. Check to see if your new patient has an order already and if the physician wants to change when they are notified.

Dr. Meister adds, "If the physician is rude that you paged them about something you had to, please let them know its policy that they are notified. Remember, we don't learn these things at all, and nurses can teach us so much here and strengthen the nurse-physician relationship in the process."

Make sure you have scratch paper handy to write down orders. You think you'll remember it, but then the physician gives you four unexpected med orders over the phone, and your CNA is trying to talk to you at the same time, and now you've forgotten them all before you've hung up. And if you work somewhere that requires you to stay on the phone with the physician while you enter orders, know that this policy isn't always realistic. Sometimes they're in a hurry, in the car, in surgery, or dealing with another very real emergency and don't have the time for you to slowly enter a nonemergent order. Be ready to quickly write something down if needed.

Don't page and then go do something else you can't stop in the middle of. Nothing makes physicians more upset than being paged, then waiting on hold for twelve minutes while you finish getting someone off the bedpan. I would be frustrated, too. I typically like to catch up on some charting or be near the desk when I page. This also enables me to have the patient's chart open if the physician asks a question that I don't know off the top of my head. If it's been over twenty minutes, page again.

Another thing to keep in mind is that they may not be ignoring your page if they don't call you back quickly. I like to compare this to when you're trying to answer a patient's call light, but then, as you're walking down the hall, somebody else needs you for something. Occasionally, you don't remember where you were going and end up totally forgetting about that original task. That happens to physicians as well. Sometimes you page while they're in the middle of something very important, and though they mean to return the page soon as they're done, something else interrupts them. So please do not assume that they're purposefully ignoring you. I know it can be easy to have that be your default thought process, as that was frequently mine.

Ask your fellow RNs if they also need to speak with that doctor. Address all of your needs simultaneously so that you're not continuing to interrupt the physician while they're seeing other patients. This will also save your coworkers some time as well; they won't have to stop what they're doing to page and wait if they know you're about to page the physician.

If they're rude, don't take it personally. The sooner you accept that, the better. Doctors get mad and rude sometimes, but that doesn't have to make you feel terrible the rest of the shift. Maybe they had a patient they were heavily invested in die earlier that day, maybe their kid wouldn't stop crying and they had just fallen asleep, or maybe they're just awful. Regardless of what's going on during their day, there is no reason for them to be disrespectful to you. Be confident and secure enough with yourself to know that if they are being rude, it's not always about you. Deal with it appropriately (either by firmly telling them not to speak to you like that or letting your manager know) and go on with the rest of your day. Their negative attitude does not get to steal your joy from you all day. It just doesn't.

Dr. Meister adds that this is especially common if you are dealing with residents: "We may be grumpy because we are working a twenty-four-hour shift and we are twenty-two hours in, or we don't understand the protocol you are following by paging. I can promise no one is the best version of himself or herself working eighty-hour weeks, but it does not excuse rude behavior to nurses."

A Lot of Cooks in the Kitchen

As you can tell, many individuals round on and care for your patient. When you start to figure in the attending physician and their support staff, multiple consulting physicians and their support staff, the team of residents, therapy services, the nursing staff, dietitians, and case managers, that alone probably equates to fifteen to twenty people.

The health care team is massive. One of the responsibilities of the bedside nurse is to help patients and their loved ones navigate through this really complex system. I find it really helpful, whenever a member of the health care team rounds, to go in with them to make sure I can hear what they're saying. This way I can continue to reinforce what they said throughout the shift with the patient. I also like to follow up after the health care team member has left to see if what they said made sense to the patient and the loved ones. I also try to notice if the health care team member does not introduce himself or herself. We get so wrapped up in our own world with our own processes that we can sometimes forget that patients don't necessarily know who we are when we walk into a room.

It took me a lot of time to put all the pieces together so that I could understand what other team members said on a level that enabled me to communicate effectively to patients and loved ones. I actually wrote another book about this, on the topic of helping patients navigate health care because it can be so confusing titled *What You Must Know When Going to the Hospital, But No One Actually Tells You.*

Remember, you are the point guard for your patient; you are the leader of the team. While the physician calls the plays, it's important for you to communicate to them if something isn't working. It's up to you to let the physical therapist know if the patient isn't stable enough to be worked with today; it's up to you to pull in the chaplain to discuss some spiritual concerns that may be inhibiting your patient's ability to make decisions; and it's up to you to talk with the pharmacist about how to optimize the timing of all of your antibiotics and balance that with your vasoactive drips into the double lumen central venous catheter.

Example of How Confident and Awesome You Can Be while Paging Physicians

RING RING!! RING RING!!

Physician (P): "This is Dr. Smith."

Nurse (N): "Hi Dr. Smith, this is Jaclyn Evans from the stroke floor. I have a question about the patient Edward Godwin in room 8123. Are you familiar with him?"

P: "No. My partner admitted him overnight and I've yet to round on him."

N: "He came in yesterday for a somewhat large left thalamic ischemic stroke. He did not receive tPA on admission. At baseline, he has right-sided weakness and numbness and tingling. Otherwise, he's been alert and oriented all day. I'm calling because he's really difficult to wake up. Before, even when sleeping, he would awaken appropriately for staff. Now, I practically have to do a sternal rub to get him to follow commands."

P: "What was his sodium this morning and how have his blood pressures been?"

N: "Sodium was 131 and it looks like he has voided approximately 5 liters in the last six hours. His latest blood pressure is 117/68. His systolic tends to run 120 to 140."

P: "Is he protecting his airway?"

N: "He started snoring, which is new, but otherwise, he's been 100 percent on room air."

P: "Get a STAT head CT scan and I'm going to transfer him to intensive care. Hopefully you can just take him straight there after the scan. You may want to call your rapid response team to assist you in case he becomes unstable."

N: "OK thanks!"

Orders you would anticipate:

- STAT BMP
- STAT head CT without contrast
- Transfer to a higher level of care

Note: If you are transferring your patient to a higher level of care, you must take the patient to the receiving unit yourself. That is the safest thing to do with a patient who is decompensating.

Chapter 6

New Nurse Basics

This next chapter is going to focus on the practical aspects of becoming a bedside nurse. I will go over report, assessments, orders, policies and procedures, documentation, and prioritization. It takes some time to get your mind around all of these concepts, let alone become efficient and finally exceptional. Remember, you are just starting out. The nurses that you're working with have a lot of experience with nursing, and have worked on that specific unit, with those specific supplies, resources, and personalities, for years. I want to reassure you: Just because it takes some time to get into the groove of things does not mean that you are a bad nurse.

Report

Ah, report.* Every unit does it a little differently, and different levels of care require different amounts of information. For example, the ED report is very short and focused, while the critical care report is extremely thorough and detailed. The floor nurses' reports are somewhat in the middle. You will get used to reporting to others on your unit, and you will also get used to

---

* **Nursepedia Definition:** *Report* is the time when nurses switch shifts and pass information to one another about the plan of care for each patient..

Elements of an Effective Report

1. **It's systematic.** You go through it the same way every single time. You always start with name, age, code status, doctors, and allergies, and you end with a list clarifying questions for the physician(s) to answer during rounds. You go through each pertinent body system one at a time. If the process is not systematic, information is often omitted.

2. **It's informative but not unnecessarily detailed.** I want to know the things about this patient that are pertinent to the next twelve hours and their overall admission. I want you to tell me the abnormals. I don't think you're a bad nurse if your report is short and concise.

3. **It quickly tells me how they came to our unit, what we're doing for them, what our plan of care is, and whether there are any emotional considerations.** I want big-picture things that I can't quickly pick out from the chart. While it's nice to know their IV access, what fluids are running, and if they're wearing sequential compression devices or not, I can already see all of that on the chart. I also like to ask the offgoing nurse if the patient and family are doing okay emotionally. I like to get a feel of the emotional climate of the room and know about the important conversations that have occurred before I go in, as that is not typically conveyed in the chart.

4. **It's uninterrupted.** When I get report, I don't ask questions until the end. If someone asks me a question while I am giving report, I say, "Hold on until I'm done and I'll answer it," because I almost always address that question in the report itself. If someone is giving you report, do not go through your report sheet asking them questions in the order in which you want to receive information. That is not how report flows. The reporting nurse tells you about the patient, and you ask clarifying questions afterward.

5. **It's considerate.** As the incoming nurse, do not spend the first ten minutes of designated report looking up information on your patients. Be considerate of other people's time. They've been here the last twelve hours; please don't make them wait because you want to look up information. If you want to know about your patient before report, you need to arrive early. Similarly, manage your time at the end of your shift so that you're not in a room doing something else you could have done earlier when report needs to start.

giving and receiving report from other units and levels of care. So if you are working in a critical care unit and receiving report from the ED, that report will be significantly shorter than a report from your unit. That does not mean it is inadequate; their focus is different. Therefore, consider where you are receiving report from and adjust your expectations appropriately.

Learning how to give an efficient, concise, yet detailed report on your unit is part of being a good nurse. Communication, my dear Watson!

I love it when someone is good at giving report. They communicate appropriately, clock out on time, and make it so that I can get started early. We all win.

I recommend keeping the same report sheet for three to four shifts before tossing it and trying a different format. I tried about three different types before I finalized the one I like. At the beginning, I would write down on my report sheet a few things I needed to remember to document in the medical record during the shift (assessment, care plan, education, telemetry strip, intake and outtake [I&O], IV, pain, etc.) so I wouldn't forget, and check them off as they were completed. During the first year, there was so much to remember to chart that these little reminders written directly on the report sheet saved me a few times, especially when I got admissions and discharges quickly.

I have my report sheet memorized, and because of that, I typically can give report completely off the top of my head and not forget anything because I can mentally go through the sheet. I actually got to the point of just using a blank sheet of paper.

Assessments

Assessments will look different depending on what unit you're working in. If you're in the post-anesthesia care unit (PACU), the ED, critical care, or hospice, your assessment may look different. Here's how to quickly rock a basic assessment for a med-surg floor patient.

Talk to your patient. Ask them questions like: What's your name? What year is it? Do you know where you are right now? How'd you get to be with me here in the hospital?

This normal conversation tells you a lot about their neurological status. It'll tell you if they're alert and oriented, if their speech is clear, and if their face is symmetrical when they talk. Don't just chitchat with them; ask them specific questions to assess their orientation status. Some patients can seem like they're really with it, and then you ask them what year it is and they say,

"Why, it's 1921, of course!" I always tell them to humor me as I ask my silly questions, so as to not insult anyone or throw them off. I proceed to ask them their name, the location, why they're in the hospital, and the month and year. (I never ask what day it is because I rarely know myself.)

Walk around their bed and see if they focus on you and track you appropriately as well.

Shine a pen light in their eye. Are their pupils equal, do they react briskly, and do they accommodate light appropriately?

Listen. Listen to their lungs in the normal six spots on their back, their heart in five spots, and then their bowel sounds in all four quadrants. Start listening in the right lower quad, which is where the ileoceccal valve (and thus the loudest bowel sound) is located.

Ask. Ask when their last bowel movement was. If it was within the last twenty-four hours, ask if it was loose or diarrhea. Many patients are on some sort of stool softener, so this will tell you if you need to hold that medication or not. However, if they are taking pain meds or are freshly post-op, make sure they get their stool softener.

Palpate. Palpate their abdomen; note if it is distended or firm and ask if there is any abdominal pain.

Grip and feel. Have them grip your hands and let go on command a few times, do a good push-pull test, and then feel their radial pulses.

Dorsi-plantar flexion and feel. Have them dorsi-plantar flex on your hands and feel their pedal pulses. I like to do this toward the end so I'm consciously not touching their feet before their hands. Gross.

Ask questions.

- "Are you having any numbness or tingling?" (Sensory assessment.) If they say yes and are diabetic, have a history of neuropathy, or always have numbness or tingling, ask if it is different than normal.
- "Are you in pain? Please rate it on a scale of 1–10." Don't forget to tell them that a 10 is burning alive or being eaten by a bear or something.
- "Do you have any questions about our plan today or anything you want to ask the doctor?" Even if they don't, I typically go over the plan anyway, then ask if they have questions after my explanation. Inevitably, I've answered a question in my explanation they didn't know they had, which sparks a whole new list of questions.

Assess the skin. It is essential that you check out their skin closely and document everything appropriately. This means checking out wounds, in between folds, bony prominences, and so on. To preserve the privacy and dignity of my younger, completely oriented patients, I wait to take a peek at their tush until the family is not in the room.

If they have any dressings that need to be changed, I wait to look and chart until I'm ready to change them, because taking tape off multiple times around a sensitive wound hurts their skin. If I'm not ready to change the dressing, I wait to look at the wound. However, use your nursing judgment. If you think it'll be hours before you can change the dressing, go ahead and peel the dressing back to take a look and replace it (unless you have an order that says not to change the dressing, as many surgeons like to remove the surgical dressing the first time). You shouldn't go a long period of time without laying eyes on the wound because it's important to ensure signs of infection are not setting in.

If they're morbidly obese or a total care patient, I wait until my certified nursing assistant (CNA) bathes them or until it's time to turn them to look at their backside. There's no need to do that right after shift change and again forty-five minutes later when they get a bath. Cluster your care and manage your time. This means that I do assessments, meds, dressing changes, and so forth at or around the time to turn them. If time permits, I typically help my CNA give baths to my patients so I can get a good look at everything on the patient, which also builds rapport with my teammates.

Always, always check their skin folds. Even thinner people have folds and we must check them because this is a common place for skin breakdown to occur. If the patient's chest is large, I'll throw a dry wash cloth on each side. That'll keep the skin dry and prevent breakdown. You must be consistent with your turns with total care and obese patients. If they develop a pressure ulcer because you didn't turn them, that's a really big deal.

Pro Nurse Tip: Use this time to also listen to posterior lung sounds if they're difficult to roll. Knock out your lung and skin assessments and turn in less than a minute.

And good Lord, do not forget to look at their heels. If they've been in bed for a while, require total care, are morbidly obese, have a poor nutritional status, and so forth, the skin on their heels can break down before you know it. It is really easy to forget about this area. I quickly lift those gams while I'm having them dorsi-plantar flex and make sure they're not getting red. If they are, toss a pillow or two underneath their shins to elevate their heels, and document that you did so (after you've documented the redness).

All the while, make sure to note if their skin is dry, flaky, pale, bruised, and so forth.

Assess lines, drains, and airways. The types of lines, drains, and airways that you will run into depends on the unit you're working on. For example, if you're in a high-risk maternity area, you most likely are not going to be dealing with ventilators or wound VACs, but if you're in a cardiac intensive care unit, you most likely will.

There are a few things to keep in mind when dealing with these devices.

First, always be aware of your hospital's policies and procedures for managing lines, drains, and airways. The policies and procedures tell you things like what you're required to document, assess, and troubleshoot, what resources are available to you, and when to notify the physician. I will discuss policies and procedures a little bit more in-depth later on.

Second, verify the information that you receive about these devices during report. For example, if the previous nurse tells me that the nasogastric tube is taped in their right nare at 78 centimeters (cm), I peek over at the patient to verify this. Patients pull out tubes, or tubes become dislodged (in some very sneaky ways!), and it can be a major issue when things are not where they need to be. I've been given a report that a patient endotracheal tube was taped at 24 cm at the lip when it was really 3 cm farther out of their mouth than reported. We had to push the tube down farther and get a new x-ray. It's helpful to assess this during report so you and the previous nurse can verify it together. Otherwise, an hour later, when you realize you're charting something vastly different than the previous nurse, you're not sure if they misdocumented the location of the tube or if it was dislodged.

Third, make sure the devices are secure. If the patient has a urinary catheter, make sure there is some sort of device that secures it to their leg (or wherever your hospital requires) to prevent the catheter from moving or being dislodged when the patient moves. It is much better to make sure these things are secured up front than to deal with them once they've become dislodged.

Fourth, know the plan related to each device. How long will the patient be utilizing it? For example, if the patient has a feeding tube, is there a plan to remove this feeding tube, or will they be discharged with it? If the patient is on a ventilator, do you have spontaneous breathing trials ordered and are they clinically appropriate for the patient? What do you need to do to get rid of this line as soon as possible? The sooner you can get rid of these things, the better.

Finally, educate. If the patient is able to understand, make sure you're explaining everything to them before and while you're doing things to decrease anxiety. Also make sure that you're educating the family or support system with the patient. A lot of these lines for tubes and airways are very concerning for people because they don't understand how they work, so the more information you can provide, the better. It's also important that they understand basic safety information related to the lines, tubes, and airways. I have had family members ask me if they could feed Bojangles to my intubated patients because they "looked hungry." Clearly, there was a knowledge deficit there about how the airway worked and how the patient was receiving nutrition. The more proactive education you can provide related to these things, the better off you, your patients, and their loved ones will be.

A drain that I am very familiar with is an extraventricular drain, which goes into a patient's brain. This drain is one where the head of the patient's bed really matters. If they improperly adjust the head of the bed, it can result in the drainage of too much or not enough cerebrospinal fluid, which, if left unattended for too long, can result in the patient's death. Therefore it's essential that you educate the patient and their loved ones that you'll be available to adjust the head of the bed and that they cannot adjust the head of the bed or the entire bed themselves. Never assume that patients and family members know about medical procedures and devices.

Many loved ones and patients may pretend they understand or nod their heads in agreement when they don't actually grasp what you're saying. If you are unsure if they understand, a good way to assess this is to just ask them a very open-ended question (for example, "Tell me what you know about this breathing tube"). Someone not having any questions doesn't always mean they understand. They may not even know the questions to ask. It is essential to ask open-ended questions and respond with understanding and grace even if they have a profound misunderstanding. We want people to feel comfortable coming to us for even the most basic and obvious questions; there are no stupid questions in health care.

The Man, the Nurse, and the Dementor Foot

It's also safe to say that, during your career as a nurse, you will encounter many ridiculous situations. You will find yourself seeing and doing things that you never dreamed you would be dealing with. I've had many of those instances throughout my career, but I would like to share a specific one with you. The mark of a good nurse is not always knowing exactly what to do every single time. It is important to be able to read a situation, identify your knowledge gaps, utilize resources appropriately, and just plain care for people. This was one of those situations I never thought I'd find myself in, and I honestly had no idea how to handle it. I never thought I would have to figure out how to deal with someone who had maggots coming out of their foot.

Yes, you read that correctly.

On one of the days I was feeling particularly confident (unjustifiably so), I was told by the charge nurse that I was going to admit a patient from the ED. This was a typical occurrence. I sat down to look at his chart on the computer before the ED called with report.

Apparently, this patient hadn't been heard from in a while so his son went to check on him at home. It had been about two weeks since he had seen him. The man was wheelchair bound, living "independently" in a pretty grotesque environment.

When his son saw him, he immediately called 911 because he "just didn't look right." EMS pulled this wheelchair-bound man out of the mess that was his home, which they later described to the ED staff as like "one of those homes on those hoarding shows."

Essentially, the patient was feeling so tired and weak that he couldn't transfer himself from the wheelchair to the toilet anymore. For whatever reason, he didn't let anyone know. During their assessment in the emergency department, they found large pressure ulcers* on the back of both of his forearms (from resting his arms on the armrests of his wheelchair) and his backside.

They had trouble finding the pulses in his feet. And, his feet didn't look good. After getting him cleaned up, he came up to our vascular surgery floor because they were concerned they would need to remove some toes, if not an entire foot. He was going to get a full workup and some additional scans and prepare for possible surgery.

The man rolled on the floor with a wonderful smile on his face that I will always remember. He was a very pleasant man and I believe he was just excited to have some company around him, even if it was the hospital staff.

---

* **Nursepedia Definition:** A *pressure ulcer* is a breakdown on the skin from extended pressure that, if not treated by removing pressure, can go down to the bone and cause extensive, irreparable damage.

Before I even introduced myself, I smelled something, something I had never smelled before, and would never, ever forget. What was that smell, you ask?

(If you've been a nurse for a while, you probably already know what's coming.)

Rotting flesh. It was rotting flesh.

Upon his arrival, the smell immediately permeated the entire room and slowly engulfed the hallway. You could smell it about four doors down from his room in either direction. It was quite literally breathtaking.

I did my typical shallow nurse breathing but could only be in the room for, at max, five minutes at a time. He was completely oblivious to it all, which did not really surprise me. This wasn't something that had happened overnight, and he had probably acclimated himself to the smell. While he was technically neurologically intact, something was off. He was aloof about what was going on, despite the emergency department staff explaining it all multiple times. I managed the first half of my assessment but had to duck out into the hallway for some fresh air. I reentered with a refreshed set of lungs.

It was now time for the last part of my assessment: the feet. I pulled off his socks, not prepared for what lay before me.

His toes were black. Not charcoal or grey. Black. Black like the dementors from *Harry Potter* black. The smell immediately intensified to a magnitude that I was not at all prepared for. I basically held my breath for thirty seconds at a time, taking two tiny breaths in between.

As I looked more closely at his toes, I thought I saw something moving. Perplexed, I leaned about as close as I could without losing consciousness, and there they were in all of their tiny, flesh-eating glory.

Maggots.

I saw two little maggots in this man's dementor foot. I had the typical "I need nurse backup" mental response and made up an excuse to immediately exit the room.

After my oxygen saturation returned to normal and my shock subsided, I slowly started to mentally process what I had seen and began to critically think about how to handle the situation. Have you ever experienced something so odd or unexpected, it feels like you're not really experiencing it? Like you're a little outside of yourself? That's how I felt as I was walking down the hall toward the nurse's station. I hadn't made any progress in my critical thinking; all I knew was that I needed the help of someone who knew more than me.

I couldn't ask just any nurse. I needed one with the strongest stomach who also knew what the heck to do in a situation like this. And I knew exactly which nurse I needed. (I'm sure all of the nurses reading this just thought of *that* nurse on your unit.) Without hesitation, she responded with everything we needed to do. I felt so reassured by her confidence. "We need to call infection control and ask them how to kill and dispose of the maggots. We need to let the attending physician know, and we need to get room spray, gowns, masks, double gloves, and whatever infection control tells us. Let's do this."

"Ok, this now sounds like a manageable task," I thought. "We will approach this in a systematic way, take care of the problem, and move on."

I felt like we were in the middle of a close basketball game. We'd just huddled for a quick time out, agreed on a plan, put our hands in the middle of the circle, said, "Go team!" and confidently walked away to destroy our tiny flesh-eating opponents.

"Let's do this," I thought in my best Will Smith in *Men in Black* voice. All I needed was some sunglasses and an isolation gown that looked like a suit.

Infection control told me to use hydrogen peroxide to kill the maggots and use a cotton-tipped applicator saturated in the hydrogen peroxide to wiggle them out. A small sealable plastic container and a red biohazard bag would be the coffin that would carry them to the incinerator located in the depths of the hospital.

I paged the physician to let him know about our stomach-churning situation. I expected him to have some elaborate orders in addition to being shocked beyond belief, as I was. I was sorely disappointed by his response. As I frantically explained what I thought was a "Stop everything you're doing, especially if you're eating, and listen to this" situation, he merely replied, "Gross," and quickly hung up.

My fellow nurse offered a few helpful hints on how to deal with the smell, because we were going to be in there until the job was done. You need to prepare appropriately if you're going to be exposed to a smell like that for an extended period of time.

We gowned up and double gloved. She dabbed the inside of our facemasks with mouthwash to combat the smell. She grabbed room deodorizer, which would only dig a small hole in this mountain of a problem, but was worth the momentary relief it provided. She also soaked small 2x2 gauze pads with mouthwash and pinned them to our gowns to provide a continual flow of fresh scent up to our nostrils, hopefully blocking any stinky air from penetrating our masks.

Her smell-prevention plan worked beautifully. We beat the insurmountable odds, withstood the odor, and removed a total of eight maggots from the man's foot, all while maintaining a calm and collected demeanor.

As I was coaxing the last maggot out from between his first and second toes, I realized that not once during this entire endeavor had I told him what was going on down there. We were so focused on the task that we forgot the essential aspect of providing nursing care: educating the patient. For all he knew, we were giving him a pedicure! He just sat there, smiling and looking around at his new surroundings.

I looked up to him as he was just sitting there, looking out the window. "Sir," I gently said, "we just removed eight maggots from your foot."

He furrowed his eyebrows with a confused look and then his face relaxed to his usual smile. "Well," he grinned, "didn't know I was feedin' a farm down there!"

Not expecting that response, I completely lost whatever train of thought I had ready to explain what we were doing and why and just stammered, "Um, uh, yes. Technically, you are correct."

Pain

Words are incredibly important in all aspects of nursing, but they are especially important when they concern pain. "Treating pain," "taking care of pain," or "getting you something to take care of your pain" mean different things to different people. It's really important to make sure you and your patient are on the same page about this; otherwise, they can have very under- or over-addressed pain. Optimizing this is a delicate balance. Managing expectations, being careful with your word choice, and communicating clearly is key to successfully addressing pain.

A patient may think that "treating pain" means you will take all pain away with a specific medication, and that if this doesn't happen, it means they need more or stronger medication. However, to the nurse, "treating pain" may mean administering a pain medication and noting a lower pain scale report. These are small and subtle yet very powerful differences.

You'll notice that health care providers talk about pain control and management, and this makes sense to us because we know that if we administered enough pain medication to eliminate all pain constantly, it could cause horrible outcomes. It's essential to ensure that the patient knows that focusing on pain *management* is our goal, not total and consistent pain *elimination*. They must understand that key difference. If patients expect you to remove all of their pain with medications and you fail to do that, they may think that you're doing a bad job and not "controlling their pain." However, if they expect some degree of pain with some medication administered to take the edge off, they will know you're doing your job appropriately, safely, and correctly.

It's important that patients know what kind of pain to be concerned about and what kind of pain is expected. For example, I expect my intubated patient to be uncomfortable, my postoperative knee replacement patient to be in pain especially when getting up, and my thoracotomy patient with a chest tube to be very uncomfortable. However, I can't just pump them full of pain medications and let them sleep all day. We have to make sure that they understand that they will experience some pain and that they need to have an understanding with the nurse about when they are creeping outside that tolerable level of pain.

At the last two hospitals I worked at, we had to ask patients on admission what a tolerable level of pain would be on a scale from 0–10. That question confused so many patients because in their minds, they shouldn't be experiencing any pain at all. It took some time and experience for me to realize that I needed to educate my patients at that specific time about realistic expectations surrounding pain.

Another piece of this whole pain management puzzle is empowering patients to appropriately describe their pain. While many of us are familiar with the "describe your pain on a scale of 0 to 10, 0 being no pain and 10 being the worst pain in the world" scale, that doesn't really give the patient a lot to go on for 1–9. And the "worst pain in the world" means very different things to different people.

Therefore, I encourage you to be able to articulate what the other numbers mean. For reference I've included a pain scale graphic.

Patients with substance use disorder

It's also important to be aware when patients who may suffer from substance use disorder are receiving pain medication. Hopefully you and the health care team will be aware of this beforehand, but the patient may not have shared this with the team. You may need to strategize a bit with the medical team about better options for pain control, because you don't want someone who is

Pain Scale

0   **No pain**

1   **Very mild:** Not noticeable, patient can function and carry on conversation

2   **Discomforting:** Somewhat noticeable, like a light skin pinch

3   **Tolerable:** Very noticeable, like stubbing your toe

4   **Distressing:** Strong, deep, and consistent, like a toothache

5   **Extremely distressing:** Strong, deep, and piercing, like when you sprain your ankle

6   **Intense:** Strong, deep, piercing, and consistent, like a bunch of insulin injections at once

7   **Very intense:** Even stronger, deeper, and more consistent pain than before, unable to be relieved, like a migraine

8   **Utterly horrific:** Childbirth contraction pain

9   **Excruciatingly unbearable:** Constant childbirth contraction pain, losing ability to maintain consciousness, pain so intense the patient may be vomiting

10 **Unimaginable:** So horrific, the patient is losing consciousness—it could not get worse, like burning alive

in recovery to get a medication whose momentary benefit does not outweigh the risk inherent to its use. However, they do need adequate pain relief. A patient suffering from a tolerance to pain medication who just had a hip surgery still needs appropriate pain relief. So how do you do this?

First, I think it's important that we are on the same page as far as definitions are concerned. Patients may have a tolerance of, dependence on, or addiction to substances. Having a *tolerance* means they need higher doses to achieve the same effects (for example, while 1 milligram (mg) of morphine may suffice for someone without a tolerance, 4 mg may be necessary for someone with a tolerance), while a *dependence* is more of an adaptive state in which, if the patient stops receiving that specific substance, they'll start to feel withdrawal symptoms. *Addiction* is very different from the previous two definitions. An addiction is when someone has a compulsion to continue to take a specific substance, has tried to stop, and has been unsuccessful in this attempt to do so. It's important to understand what specifically your patient is experiencing while you and the prescriber are coming up with a plan together.

Dealing with these situations can be really challenging, especially if you as the nurse feel that you're being manipulated. First, it's essential to understand what's going on. Are they tolerant? Are they dependent? Are they addicted? Are they recovering? It may be helpful to have some frank, open, nonjudgmental conversations with the patient first. Here's an example.

"So, typically when a patient has a pacemaker placed, it's a procedure with minimal pain involved afterward, and the pain that remains is usually controlled with oral pain medications. I want to make sure that your pain is controlled, that you're getting the support you need, and that something else isn't going on with you medically. If you don't take anything recreationally and require this much pain medication, that is a bit of a red flag that there may be a bigger problem from the surgery. I really want to make sure I know what's going on. If you've got a tolerance or dependence, that's a different matter. We can chat together about the best way to handle that, but it's really important I just know what we're dealing with so we can come up with the best plan to maximize pain control and healing."

This communicates a few things:

1. Acknowledges the elephant in the room
2. Lets them know you are meeting them where they are, not where they think they should be
3. Assures that their pain will be controlled
4. Promises that they will be supported
5. Ensures that as their nurse you care about them and will be honest with them
6. Communicates that you're on the same team

Look, if they're addicted—they're addicted. That is a very serious issue that requires specific treatment and cooperation from the patient. However, right after a major surgery, accident, trauma, or whatever else may have landed them in the hospital is most likely not the time to start this treatment. It is, however, a good time for the health care team to demonstrate honesty and empathy. If you start building trust between this person and the health care team now, you may be setting them up for success when they do agree to begin treatment for their addiction.

Again, the foundation of this is communication. You must communicate with the patient about realistic pain control and management—not pain elimination—as well as with the physician and their support staff about a plan that requires the least amount of medication and progresses the patient to discharge as fast as possible. This plan should provide enough relief to enable the patient to actively participate in their healing. And finally, by continually empathizing and building trust with the patient, you are hopefully well aware of the kind of support and needs they will have at discharge and can work with the social worker and case manager to connect them to the various community resources that can support them in recovery.

Delegation

Delegation* is an essential part of nursing. Truly, if you are carrying a full patient load, you do not have the time to provide total care to all of your patients. Tasks must be delegated to your nursing assistants (NAs) consistently and appropriately throughout your shift.

The NCLEX talks a lot about which tasks to delegate, but it doesn't necessarily tell you *how* to delegate. As a brand new nurse, how do you go about delegating to a NA who has been on this unit for fifteen years?

In the beginning of my nursing career, I would get very far behind because I was too intimidated to delegate to the NA who was sitting at the desk checking their email. I had to learn to get over my fear, delegate the task, and follow up if it wasn't completed. Truly, it's not as scary as it seems. In most cases, people are more than willing to follow through; they just can't read your mind and know what you need and when you need it. What I may have perceived as someone being unwilling to help was actually just someone killing time until their next assigned task, which they were more than willing to do.

Navigating relationships

Nursing is a little different than many other fields. You go through a lot with your coworkers, and because of that, you tend to get really close. This closeness is amazing and supportive; however, sometimes it can be enabling. At the end of the day, we're all here to take care of the patients—friendships or no friendships. We need to hold each other accountable and complete the jobs we are paid to do.

---

* I am writing this section with the assumption that you are aware of the function of a certified nursing assistant, patient care technician, licensed practical nurse, or licensed vocational nurse in your particular state. Please refer to your state board of nursing website for any questions about scope of practice.

To avoid feeling as though you are inconveniencing a friend when delegating, I recommend delegating in a matter-of-fact, all-business sort of way, using a professional tone rather than a "can you do me a favor" tone. When you present a task as a favor, you present it as something they have the option not to complete or something they don't need to prioritize over someone else's task. When you're close friends with someone, they are more willing to bend the rules, take extra time, or prioritize something else because you're their friend and would understand. I get it—it's a lot easier to ask your BFF nurse who is always helpful and nice (yet far behind) to start an IV than the grumpy nurse who floated to your unit playing on their phone at the nurse's station with the goal of doing the least amount of work possible today. However, when this becomes a consistent habit, the work and support is no longer evenly distributed, and the really nice, kind, and helpful nurse is the one who is getting dumped on or whose needs are always at the bottom of the priority list.

Please don't misunderstand me here. I understand that NAs also have a lot of tasks to complete and sometimes they do have to tell the nurse, "I'm sorry, I am absolutely swamped right now and really behind. Is there anyone else available?" I get that. I was an NA. However, that is very different from delegating a task to someone sitting in the nurse's station Snapchatting and checking Facebook. In that instance, if something is appropriately delegated, not completing the task is not an option.

Even if you're younger than your NAs, close in age, or friends, you're the nurse. It is ultimately your responsibility to ensure that tasks are completed for your patient. So when you're at work, there needs to be a certain level of professionalism maintained so your colleagues know that when you're delegating, completing the task is not optional and is their responsibility.

I know I sound kind of mean, but this is the reality of how the NA and nurse need to work together. There is absolutely no point in having NAs if nurses do not delegate appropriately. Inappropriate delegation means that you're not being efficient.

Being a nursing assistant is tough work. I worked as one during nursing school and my internship. However, just because the job isn't the easiest does not justify not delegating appropriately. When you delegate, it's nothing personal. It's not that you're trying to make someone's day tougher; it's just the job they signed up for. So if you're swamped, your patient just urinated all over their bed, and your NA is hanging out at the nurse's station, you must delegate the task to them. It can feel like you're dumping on them, but honestly you're not. Yes, you are perfectly capable of addressing that situation. However, your time would be utilized much better doing those things that only you, as the patient's nurse, can do, like passing meds, assessing, admitting, discharging, speaking with the physician,, and so forth.

Sometimes it's hard for NAs who are not in nursing school to truly understand the large number of tasks you're responsible for completing in one shift. When I was an NA, I always thought to myself, "They're complaining about charting hourly rounds, and I'm constantly charting every single thing I do! I have to chart all medications, orders, educational conversations, care plans, and changes in status, along with talking to ten different doctors, answer forty phone calls, have conversations with families, and still complete the tasks themselves as well! If only they understood."

Well, the reality is that some NAs understand and some don't. When I first started as a nurse, I worked with a great bunch of NAs. On one of my first days, I tried to stay and help clean a patient up despite the fact that I was on the verge of tears because I had so much to do that I didn't even know what to do next. I started to clean, and the nursing assistant said, "Kati, you have a million other things to do that I can't help you with. I've got this. Go." If I hadn't just met her, I would have hugged her and bought her a BFF heart necklace. (High-five, Joanna, you're awesome.)

There is an economical side to this as well. If you aren't delegating appropriately and always clock out late, while your CNAs always get out super early (because you didn't have them do anything all day), it costs more money. It's more costly to pay you overtime than to pay them their normal wages. It will also stress you out and you'll be exhausted.

Conversely, if your CNA is drowning and you're caught up, please don't spend fifteen minutes tracking them down to delegate another task that you're completely capable of taking care of independently. To be blunt, that is just really inconsiderate. Being a nurse does not mean you're above giving a bed bath, cleaning a poopy patient, walking a patient down the hall, or taking someone to the bathroom. Patient care is a team effort, so if you exclusively separate your responsibilities from the rest of your team, you alienate yourself. If you never offer support, when you are in need it will be nowhere to be found.

When I find myself delegating to someone who is not responding, I find it best to do so in a systematic, all-business kind of way.

As a side note, if someone is consistently refusing or responding very poorly when they are instructed to perform the minimal expectations, you need to speak with them about this. If after you speak with them they still refuse or respond poorly, this needs to be referred up the chain of command. It is important to hold them accountable for the job they are being paid to do. I say this because the first thing your manager will ask when you talk to them about it is "Did you talk about this with them directly?" Yes, it'll be uncomfortable to address them, but it's necessary. If this behavior is tolerated consistently, it becomes the expectation that when they show up for work, they barely have to do anything and don't have to offer support. Then the NAs who do a good job end up being asked to complete the tasks the lazy one refuses to do.

Nurse: "Sarah, can you take Mr. Smith in room 54 to the bathroom, please? Thanks."

Nurse Assistant: (Checking her schedule on the computer, no eye contact) "That's not my patient."

Nurse: "There is no one else available, and Mr. Smith needs to use the restroom. Are you saying you're not going to do that?"

Nurse Assistant: (Most likely will begrudgingly get up and go take him to the restroom)

If Sarah had said no, I would recommend further clarifying by saying something like, "So I just want to make sure I understand what's happening: you're refusing to take a patient to the restroom right now?" And if the whole *that's not my patient* mentality continues, there needs to be a chat between this NA and an assistant manager or manager about how a nursing unit functions and how the staff cares for all of the patients on the unit. During your conversation, Sarah twice refused to complete a task, which is insubordination. These are situations that need to be brought to the attention of leadership so that they can be addressed appropriately, as this behavior cannot continue.

However, people treat us as we allow them to treat us. If you delegate to someone and they respond rudely to you and you allow that, they will only continue because they know you'll take it. Not everyone has a great attitude. It can be very stressful when you are completely overwhelmed to be disrespected when attempting to lighten the load. I've truly been on the verge of tears delegating before because I did not feel empowered to respond to a bad attitude when I was overwhelmed. As much as you're able, don't tolerate people being rude to you; it is not appropriate. Remember, even though things get relaxed on the nursing unit, it is still a professional environment, and people need to be held to professional standards.

Furthermore, delegation doesn't just apply to your relationship with NAs; it applies to your nurse coworkers as well. If you're caught up and someone else is drowning, go see what you can do to help them get caught up. If you're drowning, ask someone who is caught up to help you out. There is absolutely no reason one person should be flipping through their phone at the desk while someone else is hours behind.

The entire unit is a team; it's not nurses and NAs isolated with their individual patient loads. Help each other out when it's needed. Everyone's day will run smoother if everyone knows that if things start going downhill, everyone has everyone else's back.

The response "That's not my patient" should never be spoken by an NA or a nurse. All patients on the unit are everyone's responsibility. We all watch out for one another. While patients are assigned to specific nurses and CNAs, that does not mean we should not help patients not assigned to us when it is needed. If this is the culture of your unit, I encourage you to be part of the solution. Talk to management and see if you can start a campaign with a short educational session during the next staff meeting. Turn "That's not my patient" into a bad word on the unit during the meeting. Doing so does not call anyone out specifically but does call out the behavior and change the mentality. Make it fun, so if someone says it, they have to clean all of the keyboards, put a dollar in a swear jar, restock the lab tray, or something appropriate for your unit. Do what you can to respectfully make it normal to hold each other accountable and stop unhealthy behavior.

So please, delegate gracefully. Hold each other accountable. Help out your teammates. Give great patient care. If your unit has some unhealthy ways of dealing with insubordination, delegation, or teamwork, think about solutions and be a part of them. Rock through your shift without being overwhelmed because you know your coworkers have got your back, and clock out on time.

Policies, Procedures, Order Sets, and Protocols

Regardless of where you work, you should have access to your facility's policies, procedures, and protocols. These should guide your practice at that particular institution. The last few hospitals I worked at both did a good job of explaining how to access these resources and how to practically use them at the bedside.

Basically, a policy outlines how they expect you to complete various tasks and patient care. If you don't know how to do something or how the hospital requires you to do a specific task, you should pull out that policy, read it, make sure you understand it, and then complete the task based on this policy. Many policies and procedures also have checklists that outline the order in which you are to complete specific tasks, as well as resources to look up more information about a particular task or other people to contact.

Some examples of policies and procedures include a central venous catheter removal policy, a Foley catheter insertion policy, an assessment and reassessment policy, and a restraints policy. Even years into my career, I would still pull policies if I was not sure how to do something. A few years ago, I had to give intrathecal vancomycin and could not remember all of the steps. I printed out the policy and procedure, which had a checklist attached, brought it into the patient's room, and followed it step by step as I completed the task right in front of the patient and their family. There is no shame in your policy and procedure game. If you need the step-by-step outline in front of you, use it. While it would be great to know how to do every single task off the top of your head completely accurately every single time, that's not realistic. Take whatever steps are needed to ensure you complete the task safely.

Ideally, the policies and procedures are reviewed on a routine basis by a team that includes nurses. I personally sat on a team that reviewed them during the last step before they were published, and a lot of time, thought, and consideration went into them. It was cool to see that level of care and diligence occur on the back end of bedside care. These policy decisions should always be based on the latest evidence-based practice to ensure that bedside staff are updating their care as new research becomes available. If you are interested in participating in policy review and creation, chat with your manager and see if they can point you in the right direction of who to contact to go to these meetings.

Protocols and order sets are something that I did not fully understand until I was at the bedside. Protocols are enacted by an ordering provider and include steps for the bedside nurse to follow for nursing interventions and orders. An example of a protocol would be an electrolyte replacement protocol, which is very common. If an ordering provider put in an order for this protocol, the nurse would work through the protocol, step by step, until it was discontinued.

In an electrolyte replacement protocol, the nurse will frequently have labs drawn (most likely a complete or basic metabolic panel and a magnesium and phosphorus level). Once those labs are drawn and the results are in, instead of calling the physician to order the specific replacement, the nurse can use the protocol to figure out how much of which electrolyte to replace, enabling them to enter the order themselves and administer the medication. The protocol would also indicate when to notify a physician for high and low values, when to recheck lab values, and any other considerations.

These protocols enable you to work autonomously so you're not constantly calling a physician or their support staff for orders. It also frees up the ordering providers to focus on other things than standardized care. It's important that you're very familiar with the protocol itself so that you're not missing an important step.

Protocols can be very basic and straightforward, or they can have many steps. I've personally had experience with the following protocols: sepsis, withdrawal of life support, heparin, anemia, stress ulcer prophylaxis, deep venous thrombosis prophylaxis, electrolyte replacement, and more. The physician or their support staff will enter an order for the protocol itself, and then the nurse takes it from there, notifying them when appropriate.

While protocols are wonderful, they're definitely not a one-size-fits-all kind of situation. They work for most, not all. Therefore, if there's something going on with your patient that makes you concerned about putting them on a specific protocol, chat with the prescriber about it. Also, if you see a provider coming by and ordering things on a patient that may conflict with an ongoing protocol, it's essential to clarify the situation with them. Once, I had a patient on an electrolyte replacement protocol, and I was ordered to give a total replacement of 80 milliequivalents (mEq) of potassium over the day. The nephrologist rounded, saw the low potassium in the labs, and ordered another 80 mEq, not seeing that I already had a protocol running that addressed the hypokalemia. I had to call the nephrologist to clarify, who then told me to discontinue the order he just placed. Make sure you are critically thinking before implementing orders, especially when working with protocols and various providers.

I've heard physicians refer to protocols as having an 80/20 rule, meaning they work for about 80 percent of patients and don't work for about 20 percent. Having been exposed to protocols as a new grad and throughout my entire career at the bedside, I think that's a pretty accurate estimation.

Pro Nurse Tip: If you're working at a teaching hospital with residents or with a new physician, don't always assume they have the protocols memorized backward and forward. Help them out, or let them know if the patient wouldn't be appropriate for that particular protocol.

Order sets are a little different than protocols. Many hospitals come up with order sets based on disease processes, like stroke, myocardial infarction, heart failure, kidney failure, suicide attempts, and many more. This is something that hopefully the physician or their support staff fills out once a patient is admitted with a particular issue. On their screen, it populates a bunch of standard orders for a patient admitted with that particular issue.

For example, let's say a patient was admitted with a stroke and the admitting provider is filling out the stroke order set. This order set will contain all of the necessary orders a typical stroke patient may require: things like a follow-up CT scan, follow-up labs, aspirin, blood pressure medications, some sort of deep venous thrombosis prophylaxis, a diet order, a swallow study, physician and occupational therapy, or a consult to case management.

As a bedside nurse, I really loved order sets because I essentially had all of the orders I needed. I didn't have to call a physician in the middle of the night for a simple diet order or a swallow study. However, the challenge with order sets is that providers may just fill out the order set and not necessarily address all of the patient's needs. People can get really into the order set mindset, thinking that everything will be on there, when it isn't necessarily. Again, thinking critically is key.

Documentation

Oh, documentation. I have such a love-hate relationship with documentation. It's very necessary, but also very frustrating. I have a few tips for you as you're learning the documentation requirements of your specific facility.

Pay close attention in your documentation classes during orientation. Look for ways to be faster at charting. Keep in mind: This doesn't mean you're charting less; you're just being more efficient with it. Pay attention for shortcuts or tips and tricks about how to navigate the system faster, as well as how to avoid unnecessary documentation..

Take a look at your facility's policy regarding documentation expectations. It helps to know what's expected of you, so you're not under-charting or over-charting.

Just because it was documented doesn't mean it was done. I'm sure you're very familiar with the phrase, "If it wasn't documented, it wasn't done." However, I have seen people copy and paste documentation to meet the documentation requirements while not actually performing the task on the patient. Therefore, it's important to know that you should only document the things that you physically do and see. Never document ahead of time, never document for someone else, and never document something you did not physically do just to fill in all the boxes or meet minimum requirements. I think people equate not doing all the little things they need to do every single shift with failure. Honestly, it's not realistic to complete hourly rounding on seven patients, be on time with all meds, admit and discharge, administer pain meds and follow up on all of them, take and chart vitals exactly when they are due, and so forth. Even really experienced nurses miss stuff on some days. An emergency occurs and they miss an hourly round or two, or a med is late. Do not get so sucked into this concept of perfect documentation that you're documenting things that are not actually true.

Document like it will be read in a deposition in five years. It is important to paint a very good clinical picture with your documentation. Try to have the mentality that you will look at this chart five years from now never having thought about it since and will, all of a sudden, have to understand exactly what happened that shift. You think you'd remember things later, but after a while, all of them sort of blend together.

I have participated in chart reviews over the years when a sentinel event occurred, and we were looking back to see what exactly was going on with the patient throughout their stay. One thing that was pretty consistent regardless of the unit, hospital, or people was the poor quality of documentation. It is really important for someone to be able to look at what you have documented during your shift and be able to understand specifically what was going on with the patient at that time.

For example, if a patient went into rapid atrial fibrillation with rapid ventricular response, causing you to initiate a Cardizem drip, after which the patient was transferred to another unit, you are not only responsible for documenting starting the drip but the calls to their physicians, the physicians' responses, updates in the plan of care, communication with patients and loved ones, and even that you gave report to the next nurse.

If it seems like there's a lot to constantly consider throughout your shift, it's because there is. Getting all of this to become not only part of your normal thought processes, but also fluidly incorporated into everything you do will take time. It's kind of like learning how to drive. At first, everything seems scary, new, and important, but after a while, you learn about the priorities and what doesn't quite matter as much, as well as how to handle tough situations. In time, you learn how to drive on the interstate, in heavy traffic, through the mountains, or in rain, sleet, or snow. Soon, driving becomes second nature.

You know what you're doing and could practically do it with your eyes closed. But it is important to always remain cautious and aware of your ability to do harm. A careless nurse is just as capable of harming people as someone who texts behind the wheel is. And as new technologies develop, the responsibilities of the nurse increase, much like the person using Snapchat while driving. The potential for fatal harm in the absence of diligence is profound.

Chapter 7

Time Management

I'd like to describe a scenario that is painfully familiar for many new graduate nurses.

You've just started your new job on a med-surg floor. You have a great preceptor, you like your unit, and your manager seems pretty cool. But you dread going to work.

You get report and you're already an hour behind. You're overwhelmed. There are so many things to do right that second that you shut down. You can't do this. It's too much. You struggle through each day just trying to get to the end of the shift. You are elated for days off. You dread going back. Is this really what you signed up for? Will this *ever* end?

Sound familiar?

Been there. Felt that. And I want to tell you that yes—dear Lord, yes—it does get better. I also want to tell you some ways to work through this because you can do this.

Let me repeat myself.

You can do this.

You may have heard of the term "time management" before in school. While it sounds very general in school, it's an incredibly necessary aspect of being a successful nurse.

As a nurse, you are responsible for completing, charting, and monitoring a great deal within a shift. Because of this, you have to know how to appropriately manage your time to get it all done. If you don't, you'll never clock out. You'll just live at the hospital, and before you know it, you'll be a patient.

Time management is not just another good concept to be aware of; you will not survive without it. I like to compare this (along with most other things) to Harry Potter. Harry does have magical powers (were any of you *meant* to be a nurse or felt called to this profession?) and a foundational magical knowledge (hello, nursing school), but to get things done, he must know his wand.

Wands are what connect the power and knowledge to physically getting things done. It is the same with time management. You can know all of the theory, pathophysiology, and pharmacology in the world, but if you don't know how to manage your time, you will be chasing your tail all day and that wonderful and thoughtful care you wanted to provide will not happen. If you're not using time management, your patients won't receive timely care, you will miss important clinical information in the shuffle, and you'll burn out faster than a Samsung cell phone.

Time management is to nursing what Harry's wand is to his spellcasting. It gets things done.

A few key aspects of time management are delegation, prioritization, and intuition. There are also some important principles to keep in mind as you're developing your own style.

Please know that while it would be wonderful if there were a correct and an incorrect way to go about time management, it's not that cut and dry. Everyone has their own style. While some may do things in a slightly different order, what matters is that things are being addressed as clinically appropriate, patients' needs are being met, the nurses are caring for themselves, and policies and procedures are being followed.

In the wizarding world, everyone's wand is different and every witch or wizard has their own style to their magic. Time management in nursing is the same.

I would like to now shine a light into the abyss of uncertainty about time management for those of you that are just now being exposed to it. So, in true Potter form: *Lumos!*

(For all of you Muggles out there, the Lumos spell creates a beam of light from the end of a wand. Too perfect, right?)

A few important aspects of time management include general etiquette, delegation (which we discussed in the previous chapter), prioritization, key principles, and intuition. I will discuss each of these, along with time management tips and sample timelines specifically for the nursing floor and critical care environments.

General Time Management Etiquette

Remember, nursing care is a continual process. While we would all like to hand off and receive our patients with all tasks completed and in the best shape possible, that's not realistic. Patients deteriorate, admissions arrive, and codes always seem to happen around shift change. (My first child was a shift change baby.) You may clock in one day and find that you have five new orders you need to implement right away that were put in twenty seconds before shift change started.

It is not appropriate for the previous nurse to stay late to implement orders they could not complete in the time allotted. That's just not how being part of a team works. However, this is not a hard rule. It's important to understand that if you're getting report and see there were a set of new orders placed just before shift change, you'll most likely be responsible for implementing them. The previous nurse should do their best to complete what's possible, but there is absolutely no reason for them to stay late.

Therefore, if you're getting ready to clock out in twenty minutes and a new admit rolled in the door fifteen minutes ago, you do your best to get as much done as possible. However, the oncoming nurse should not expect you to stay an extra hour to get the admission orders completed. Please, don't become that nurse who acts like people are lazy for not completing tasks that weren't their responsibility in the first place. Complete your work and do not try to pawn it off on the next nurse.

Spoiler alert: Everyone hates that nurse. Don't become them.

If we all have similar expectations, then people don't end up feeling short-changed or taken advantage of. There will be days when you start out implementing unexpected orders and other days you don't have to. This goes back to what I discussed in chapter 1 about good nurses. Sometimes, people—including coworkers—are so focused on their task list and their needs that they forget about the other people around them. While it's not fun to start your day with a bunch of new orders, it's also not fun to have such an insane shift that you didn't even have a chance to start them. Communication is essential in these instances, especially if your coworker clearly has different expectations than you.

Again, nursing is a continual process in a constantly changing and unpredictable environment. Nurses should not expect to start their shift exactly the same each day—this is an extremely dynamic field. You never know what you'll be walking into! The more flexible you can be, the better off you will be.

If you feel the previous nurse left you with too much to do and clearly had time to do it, address it before they leave and don't complain to the entire nurse's station about how lazy they are. I encourage you to ask them to complete whatever missing tasks need to be addressed in a very matter-of-fact (not snarky) tone. Examples could be:

- "Oh, and if you could hang a new bag of Levophed before you leave, that'd be great. Thanks."
- "Can you give that heparin shot that was due at 0600 before you take off? Thanks."
- "Their blood sugar was due an hour ago; if you could grab that before you leave, I'd really appreciate it."

However, use judgment. You want to help out when things are crazy. If you know a nurse has had a terrible shift and they're going to be staying late to chart anyway, help them out and just take care of those things. But if you're walking on the unit and the previous nurse is hanging out at the nurse's station sipping coffee and checking their phone, clearly there was time to take care of their basic responsibilities. Some people just need a gentle reminder. This is essential: You want to be caring and helpful, but you do not want to be a pushover.

Again, patient care is dynamic and things change quickly. Therefore, it's important to extend a lot of grace, understanding, and support to your coworkers. However, some people try to take advantage of this so they can do the least amount of work possible. Please do not turn into the nurse whose personal goal is to do the least amount of work during each shift. If you are a nurse with this mentality, you are the dementor of the unit: You are sucking the life out of your coworkers. People leave nursing units because of coworkers like this. Nothing frustrates people more than coworkers who complain about normal aspects of the job that they signed up to do.

Finally, if a coworker does bring something to your attention that maybe you missed or calls you out on something you knowingly did not do, own up to it, correct it, and move on. Do not take it personally. Being able to call each other out on things when we knowingly or unknowingly mess up is absolutely critical. It's uncomfortable, but we have to be okay with that uncomfortable space. If someone respectfully and privately calls you out on something or you do that to someone else, do not treat them differently afterward. It is not personal. You're just professionals practicing professional accountability with one another, and graceful, professional accountability, understanding, and teamwork are the foundation of an amazing nursing unit.

Prioritization

Prioritization is a key aspect of time management. You have to figure out what is the most important thing to do, and the next thing, and the next thing, and the next thing. What most people think about when they hear the word is how to prioritize your tasks on your own. However, there is another aspect of this: verbalizing this prioritization to other people. Now, I don't mean that you have to tell everyone what you're doing at every point in the day. What I mean by this is that when ten people come up to you with things that need to be done this moment, how do you communicate in a nice way to someone that what they need is not your priority? That was a challenge that I did not realize existed until I was faced with it.

Many people will act like absolutely everything is a priority right this very second (from therapy, to management, to the doctor, to the physician assistant, to the radiology tech, to the family member), but you as the nurse must look at your task list and prioritize everyone else' priorities.

You must think to yourself: "Everything is a priority to everyone. I need to decide what the priority is for me and my patients right now. I am the nurse, the common denominator. I see the big picture. Now, what needs to be done first?"

I feel like a lot of my day is reassuring people and calming them down because things don't happen as quickly as they would like them to. It is totally okay to make people wait when appropriate. You're the nurse and you're the one whose time is absolutely precious. (I am not saying other people's time is not, but you are the gatekeeper for your entire patient load and can only do one thing at a time for each of them.)

Remember: You, no one else, get to dictate what order you will do things.

Your patient's mother may be livid that the scheduled Colace is ten minutes late on her fifty-four-year-old son who is being discharged today, but she doesn't know that your other patient next door just flipped into atrial fibrillation with rapid ventricular response and a heart rate of 167.

I am a big fan of talking points, because sometimes I know I need to communicate something simple, but I don't know how to put it simply. Here are a few suggestions for how to nicely tell people that what they want you to do right this second will not be done any time soon.

- "I hear that you need _____ right now, and I will address that as soon as I finish with this priority. Thanks for letting me know."
- "I have some very pressing patient needs right now. I will get to that as soon as humanly possible."
- "Thank you for letting me know—I will be there as soon as I can, after I'm done taking care of what I'm dealing with right now."

Using a calm, reassuring tone, communicate with people as they come to you with things they need addressed. As you become more experienced, you'll be able to deal with more at a time and prioritize faster.

The other aspect of prioritization is ordering your tasks. I'll talk more about that later on, but an important part of it is determining the urgency level of everything. Is this a "drop everything right this second" or a "this patient will decompensate without immediate intervention" kind of situation, or do you have a little wiggle room?

Let me give you an example. When a new nurse gets an order to transfuse blood, they may think that they need to drop everything and go do that immediately because = new and scary. However, think about the *reason* they're getting blood. Is it because of acute blood loss or asymptomatic anemia? Or are they chronically anemic, have a hemoglobin level that has slowly dropped over the last few days, and now are finally getting a transfusion because it's just below normal?

Acute situations mean you do need to drop everything. Chronic, proactive situations and orders mean you can get a few more important things done first. If you get an order for a unit of blood for a chronically anemic and asymptomatic patient while it's mid–med pass, and you've got two patients left with insulin due with their trays in front of them, you should quickly finish those two meds before ordering your blood.

Things that seemed like acute or drop-everything tasks in school may not be on your unit. For example, in school, if a central line dressing needed to be changed, a blood pressure medication needed to be given, or an IV pump was beeping, those were drop-everything scenarios. Not so much in the real nursing world.

As you gain more experience on your unit with your specific patient population, you'll learn different levels of urgency. What may be a drop-everything situation on one unit may not be on another.

To summarize, communicate effectively with people when they present you with a new task that needs to be prioritized, and be able to differentiate between acute or drop-everything needs and chronic or proactive needs.

General Time Management Principles

Let's go over a few important things to keep in mind as you are learning time management, regardless of the unit you're working on.

Take your thoughts captive

When you are already overwhelmed and defeated before you've even clocked in, it's important to stop those thoughts before they take over. This doesn't just apply to the overwhelmed new graduate nurse; this applies to anyone who struggles with a self-defeating attitude. We can be our own worst enemy at times, and it's important to stop that thought process before it takes over. This is a very active process.

Identify when you get down on yourself the most or begin to feel that hot, overwhelming feeling creep up your chest to your face. Maybe it's before you clock in, during your drive to work, after you get report, or while you're on the phone receiving report on your first admission. When you start to feel it, remind yourself that you can do this.

Yes, you.

You can do this.

If there are thoughts trying to creep in, and your brain is going over all of the worst-case scenarios, creating those fictitious arguments with others that you inevitably lose, or imagining problems that aren't there, actively tell those thoughts, "No, that is a lie. I can do this. I can handle this."

Take a deep breath. Do some Rocky Balboa air punches. Shake off the nerves.

And bring. It. On.

Tackle your tasks with a plan

Identify the routine tasks, like scheduling medications, turns, assessments, and documentation, and also the nonroutine tasks that you're dealing with today.

Maybe you've got a patient who's heading off to dialysis in the next twenty minutes and needs their meds, so you know you have to see them much sooner than everyone else. Maybe two physicians are rounding at the same time and a patient needs pain medications right now, or maybe you've already gotten discharge orders from that surgeon who rounds at 0600 every day.

Now that you've identified these things, how can you weave the nonroutine stuff with the routine stuff? Can you go grab the dialysis patient's medications, quickly administer them, and complete a speedy assessment before they head off the unit? (Bonus if you can chart that assessment in the room really quickly as they roll out of the room.) Can you round with those physicians and complete part of your assessments while you're in the rooms with them?

Weaving nonroutine into routine is how you consolidate tasks, deal with the expectedly unexpected, and manage your time like a rock star.

Managing your time when everything is urgent

It never fails. You start your day with the best intentions. You begin your assessments and meds on time (woo-hoo!), and then all of a sudden three doctors round at once and expect you to implement their orders immediately. One patient needs to pee, one needs pain meds, lab is on the phone with an alert lab value, a family member is on the phone waiting for an update, and the STAT med you called for an hour ago hasn't shown up yet.

Good. Lord. What do you do now?

While this may seem like an extreme example, it's not, because you already spend all day prioritizing and reprioritizing. When you think you have your next two hours figured out, something inevitably comes up. The key is being able to reprioritize in an instant. I will tell you what I do when suddenly everything is urgent and I have no clue what to address first.

First, stop and take three deep breaths. Recollect yourself. Don't just go— you need a plan to maximize your time. A wise patient once told me, "When things start to get serious, the first pulse you take is your own."

Second, think about which patient is the least stable and address them first. Please keep in mind this is not always the one complaining the loudest. While one patient may be extremely upset that it's taken forty-five minutes to get them their 4 mg IV morphine, your other patient, who just had a graft placed and has a blood pressure of 192/91, is your priority.

Third, what can you delegate? If a patient needs to void and a nursing assistant is available, delegate. If a patient needs pain medication and you know another nurse is caught up, ask if they can give the med for you. Nursing is a team sport. We all are taking care of the entire unit together. That means when you're caught up, you're helping others who are behind. Trying to do everything on your own when others are caught up is a disservice to yourself and your patients. You will be running ragged and it will take forever to get your patients' needs addressed. Working together as a team is an essential part of a well-functioning and safe nursing unit. I know it can be hard to ask others to help you, but please do. Most are more than willing to help.

Fourth, what can you do simultaneously? If a family member is on the phone wanting an update but you also need to see what meds you can give another patient, look that up while you're on the phone. Whenever I'm on the phone and anticipate being on hold, I always get by a computer and chart or look things up simultaneously. Consolidating tasks, trips, phone calls, and so forth is essential. When you see a patient, always ask if there's anything else they need before you leave. It's incredibility inefficient to be with a patient and try to leave immediately without first asking if they need anything else, because they will inevitably put on their call light seven minutes later for something you could have addressed while you were in the room.

Fifth, remember that charting is the last priority. If you do have a second, chart the random or difficult to remember thing, but this matters the least in busy moments. Always chart your medications in real-time, but charting assessments can wait when you're that far behind. Make notes if you need to, but when you're running from an unstable patient to a new admission to a screaming discharge, charting is going to have to wait.

Sixth, apologize for being late to patients and families. Never respond with excuses—they don't help the situation (honestly, they can make it worse). Provide a heartfelt apology, even if it was not your fault. Knowing that you are truly sorry for taking so long to get their pain medication (even though you were hanging blood, rounding with an upset physician, and giving an antihypertensive med for a patient with a BP of 238/104) means quite a bit to people. Additionally, apologizing immediately can smooth things over before they get rough. Having a grumpy patient or family can make the shift tough.

I have spoken with many nurses over the years who express concern with apologizing to patients and families. Many equate apologizing with an admission of guilt, like you did something wrong and could be held liable. I can definitely empathize with that concern, being very protective of my nursing license and not wanting anything to jeopardize it; however, never apologizing when simple things are missed or require acknowledgment is a disservice to our patients. Missing an hourly rounding because you were tied up with a decompensating patient, forgetting your patient requested to speak with you, or ordering the wrong meal tray are legitimate reasons to offer a simple apology.

If you are concerned about apologizing, I highly recommend speaking with your manager and asking specifically how to handle it. Apologizing is an important aspect of patient satisfaction. You're not perfect, you or another member of the health care team will mess up sometimes, and you, as the nurse, will be at the bedside all day; what matters is that you handle it in a professional manner, which includes acknowledging mistakes sometimes.

I have included an example of an effective apology.

Effective Apology

- **Instead of:** "Sorry it's taken so long for me to get here. We're so short-staffed today it's not even funny!"

  Why this is not great: Technically you're apologizing, but you're also telling them there's not enough staff to quickly address call lights. While that may be true, it will make your patient and their family uneasy and nervous, which won't help your situation.

- **Try:** "I'm really sorry it took a while for me to get your medication. How have you been feeling? Is there anything I can get for you while I'm here?"

  Why this is better: You apologize and acknowledge their concern and frustration immediately and quickly center everything on how they are feeling and how you can satisfy their needs.

I know it's really frustrating to be short-staffed and drowning all day. I've definitely been there and it's pretty overwhelming, even for experienced nurses. However, it's not the patient's fault that three nurses called out and we couldn't get the NAs we need, so simply apologizing to them is the best approach. That frustration and need should be directed toward management, staffing, or whoever would be appropriate in your facility—not the patient, even if they are really upset.

Even though I've been a nurse for a while, I still have to remind myself of these things. Sometimes I get overwhelmed and can't figure out what to do next and have to remind myself to stop and go through the steps. Occasionally, I have to talk to a coworker: "OK, I'm really overwhelmed and I'm not sure what to do next right now. Could you help me think this through?" Just talking through it out loud to someone else helps me focus and figure out my priorities.

An example

Background: Let's say you're working on a med-surg unit and you are caring for six patients.

Situation: You are giving meds to your second patient. He starts to puke. You look into your computer chart and see an order for two units of blood on your first patient and an order for Zofran on your puking patient. On your way to get Zofran from the Pyxis, a family member calls and wants an update on your third patient. A doctor is rounding and starts asking questions about your fourth patient. While the doctor is asking questions, your fifth patient is on their call bell because they need to go to the bathroom and want a pain pill for a mild headache. Oh, and a family member of your sixth patient says they are really, really lethargic and breathing weird all of a sudden.

Now that you're short of breath from reading that, in what order do you do everything?

Plan: First, take a deep breath. Second, put your Nurse Face on because you can handle this.

Talk to the doctor while walking to the Pyxis to get the Zofran.

Have whoever answered the phone with the family member of the third patient take a message—you'll call in thirty minutes.

Ask the nurse who just discharged three patients, is all caught up, and is flipping through her phone in the nurse's station to give the Zofran you just pulled. Tell her the patient is currently puking.

Delegate to your tech checking her email to get a set of vitals on your sixth patient, and make sure to tell the tech that this needs to be done now, because the patient is having changes. Tell her to take your fifth patient to the bathroom when she's done, and have her tell them that you'll be there in ten minutes with a pain pill.

Go check on your sixth patient who just got a fresh set of vitals. Call the doc, if needed. While you're waiting for the doc to respond, fill out your blood request form, and grab the pain pill from the Pyxis. Wait to send the blood request down until you hear from the doc about your sixth patient. You want to make sure there aren't any STAT orders you need to complete because once you send for the blood, it's on its way, and you'll only have thirty minutes to hang it (and you have to be in the room for the first fifteen minutes).

If everything is good with your sixth patient, send down your blood request form, and while they're working on sending the blood, give your pain pill. (Bonus: You know they have three other meds due in fifteen minutes, so you snag those as well.) If your blood isn't there by the time you get done with that, call the family member back and check to see if the Zofran worked on your second patient.

You've put out six fires. And it's only been twenty-eight minutes.

Time Management on the Floor

I learned time management well when I worked on an acute-care nursing step-down with cardiac, vascular, and stroke patients. I typically had four to five patients on day shift and five to six on night shift. Report happened twice, was thirty minutes long, and ended at 0730 and 1930. On day shifts, I'd wrap up charting at 1030, and on night shifts, at 2300 (assuming I didn't get an admission or have a patient decompensate during that time). First, I'm going to over some general time management tips and then I'll go into a general timeline.

1. **Maximize report.**

Seek out the person you're getting report from and get started right away. Don't waste time. The longer you hang out at the nurse's station sipping coffee, the further behind you'll be. Complete report at the bedside so that you can actively verify information while it is being verbalized by the previous nurse.

While the previous nurse is going through report, learn how to take report quickly:

- Use abbreviations as much as possible
- Customize your own report sheet so you're not rewriting the same things over and over again

- Only write pertinent information
- Don't get caught up in filling out every little box on your sheet
- Use a pen you like because that's always fun

Before you leave the room, introduce yourself to the patient, ask them if they need anything, and tell them when to expect you back. If you address immediate needs and provide a timeframe for when you'll be back, you'll cut down on those shift change call lights.

Example: "Alright Mr. Jones, I am going to get report on my other patients now. Is there anything I can grab for you? I'll be back in about an hour to bring some medications and do my assessment."

Pro Nurse Tip: If they are a patient who has had pain, ask them to rate their pain at this time and see if they need any medication for it. That way you can bring it in when you planned to come back, instead of having to make an additional trip out of the room and back when they request it.

2. **If family members call for an update during or shortly after shift change, tell them (or the person who answered the phone) that you will call them back once you have assessed the patient and introduced yourself.**

That kind of nonemergent stuff can wait until you see what kind of shape all of your patients are in. You'll also be able to give them a better update after you have fully assessed their loved one and read the chart.

3. **Start with your least time-consuming patient first, then progress to your more time-consuming patients, seeing the most time-consuming patient last.**

Take a look at all of your patients collectively and think about which patient will take the longest to provide care to at the beginning of the shift. Many times, nursing units will assign patients to nurses based on how much care they require (drips, drains, airways, isolation precautions, tube feedings) so that one nurse doesn't have a bunch of patients who require little assistance while another has all total-care patients.

Figure out which of your patients will take the most time and plan to see them last. Then, look at the rest of your patients and create a plan of what order you will assess and medicate them. It's not the end of the world if you could have ordered them differently, and there isn't a right or wrong way to order them, but I have found this to be the most efficient method. Things may also change as you're moving. Maybe one patient put on his call light and wants some pain medications, so you just grab the rest of his meds and do it all at once. This may change your original order, but as long as it's getting done at some point, that's what ultimately matters.

Things to consider when developing this order:

- *The amount and route of medications:* Are there just four pills, or are there two pills, two intravenous piggyback (IVPB) antibiotics, an IV push med, and a suppository? Do you need to crush and flush them all down a feeding tube?

- *Time-sensitive meds:* Insulin is a big one for a day shift. Sometimes, patients' time-sensitive meds dictate the order in which you should see them.

- *Any other nursing care necessary at that time:* Do you need to perform dressing changes, total care turns, enteral feedings, and so forth?

- *How talkative the patient or family is:* Seriously, I have seen some patients later or last because I knew they would want to chit-chat, and I simply didn't have time because I needed to see my other patients.

- *If you need help turning them to assess them:* If I had a total-care patient and needed help to assess their backside and posterior lung sounds, I would touch base with my nursing assistant and see when they'd have time to go in the room with me to knock their care out at the same time.

You would rather be late on one patient's medications than be late on four or five patients' medications. After you decide which patient will take the most time, peek into their room and say something like, "I'll be in to give your medications and complete an assessment in about an hour or so. I am just going check out my other patients first so I can spend more time in here later. Is there anything I can get you right now?" By stopping in their room and letting them know you'll be back, you give them a timeframe to work with, and you can address any immediate needs to prevent a call light while you're seeing your other patients.

4. **If able, chart in the patient's room right after you complete your assessment or care.**

This cuts down significantly on interruptions. Charting in the hallway or nurses' station is extremely inefficient because of the number of times you'll be interrupted. If you're in the room with the patient, you can chart faster.

Also, if you forget to ask them something or check something, like a wound, then you can quickly do that and chart it.

If you can't chart your entire assessment in the room, chart only the things that are different or abnormal. Go back later when you have time to fill in the stuff that is normal or the items that are same for most patients. This creates a timestamp for when you were in the room. You'd be surprised how quickly you forget information.

It can be a little awkward to stand at a computer and chart silently while the patient is sitting in their bed next to you, but I encourage you to get used to it! People appreciate your presence, even if you're not engaged in a ton of conversation. Please do not feel like you can't take the time you need to enter important information into their chart. It ensures the best accuracy if you're charting information while you're in the room with that specific patient. Information sort of blurs together when you have multiple patients.

It can get confusing if you're waiting until you see everyone to chart everything. Rarely will you get that amount of uninterrupted time to chart that much information. I've tried this on multiple units and it's never worked. I always ended up behind, finding myself charting information from 0900 at 1700 or later. I repeat—do not see all of your patients first, and then attempt to chart all at once. If you're pressed for time, while you're in the room, chart the small amount of abnormal information so that you will at least have something to jog your memory.

5. **Save your nonemergent or nonurgent questions for when the doctor rounds.**

Things that may have seemed like an emergency in nursing school aren't as much of an emergency in the real world. You don't need to drop everything and page the doctor at 0740 because you have a question about a med due at 1100. It'll take a little time to adjust your urgency level from the very general things you learned in school to what's necessary to know and apply on your particular unit and patient population. Nursing school teaches you to notify the physician in many different scenarios, but it's important to learn how soon you actually need to notify them. There are a few occasions in which it is as soon as possible (critical lab values, changes in status, and other high-priority concerns), but generally speaking, many things can wait for rounds. This saves you time, as you're not stopping to page and get a call back at inconvenient times, and it also saves time for whomever you are paging.

6.   **Don't go do something else in the middle of passing medications.**

Someone may say, "Hey, can you help me get Ms. Matthews on the bedpan real quick?" while you're scanning your meds. Don't do it; this is when medication errors occur. Let them know you're in the middle of passing meds to a patient, and once you're done, you'll help them. Trust me, it's pretty tempting to stop what you're doing and help, but do your best to focus during these times.

7.   **Knock out your meds, assessment, and charting all at once.**

I know it's not always possible, but this is the most efficient way of completing care. For this to work, you have to be able to quickly and efficiently utilize your charting system. I like to walk into the room, put my meds down, and then assess my patient. Then, I'll scan all of my medications, and while the patient is working on taking their meds, I'll chart my assessment. The information is fresh, you have some time to build rapport with the patient and family, and you don't have to worry about finding time later to document what you just did. Also, if you are going through your documentation and realize you missed something, you can immediately address it rather than having to come back later. Once you get used to the charting system, you'll be able to input an assessment in under three minutes if you put effort into learning how to do it in a systematic, efficient way.

Floor Nursing Timeline

Let's say I'm walking around, getting report on my five patients. During report, I introduce myself, give them a quick run-down of the day, and let them know that I'll be back to bring meds and do my assessment soon. This should sound something like this:

"Hi, my name is Kati and I'll be your nurse today. Today, we have an MRI scheduled, and it looks like I'll be drawing some blood around lunchtime and again around dinner. I'll explain a little bit more about the MRI later. If those labs come back where we need them to be, we could be looking at discharge tomorrow. I'll be back in about thirty to forty minutes to bring some more morning medications and do an assessment. Is there anything you need right now?"

This implies that you'll be back so they shouldn't ask you for anything immediately in a polite way that lets them know you still care about them but have a lot to do. When you communicate with your patients and families, you cut down on call lights asking to see you just to ask a question. Maximize that time at the bedside with thorough communication.

I make a quick exit because I have a lot of care to coordinate for the five patients I currently have in addition to the two I'll probably receive this afternoon. Then I run back to the nurse's station (hopefully before anyone needs anything) and see who has 0730 or 0800 meds or breakfast insulin and say hello to my nursing assistants. Addressing your NAs should sound something like this:

"Hey Travis and Denessa, how are you today? Gah, that Starbucks looks delicious. I had a white chocolate mocha yesterday. Yum. Anyways, the guy in room 73 uses the urinal but needs help or else we'll have ten total bed changes on our hands, 82 is a high fall risk who almost fell last night, and 83 will be discharged early today. Let me know when you're giving baths and I'll try to help."

Delegation is also important at this busy time. If you're giving meds or assessing and the patient needs something that will take more than three to seven minutes, delegate this task to the nursing assistant if they are available. This may sound inconsiderate, but you honestly do not have time. You should spend approximately fifteen minutes with each patient between charting and meds. If you spend twenty to twenty-five minutes with each, you'll be late on your meds. I used to essentially provide total care at the beginning of my shift because I felt bad delegating. I ended up being with all of my patients for thirty to forty-five minutes each. It simply doesn't work and ends up being more inefficient. Delegate in a non-jerky, all-business kind of way.

I analyze my patient list and consider all variables listed in the previous section when deciding who to see first. I grab their meds and go. As stated before, I get whatever I need before heading into the room. I assess, then scan meds, then chart while they are taking their meds. Before leaving the room, I ask if they need anything before I leave and let them know I'll be back to check on them in roughly one to two hours, after I've checked on my other patients.

This timeline, without interruptions, should get you done with all charting and meds by 1000 or 1015.

Time Management in Critical Care

Critical care nursing is very different from floor nursing. It is less task management and balancing for multiple patients and more in-depth, big-picture thinking on two patients. The stakes are a bit higher, as patients are unstable, and practically everything is time-sensitive. Your stress level is high, not because you have a lot of tasks to complete, but because people are acutely decompensating and it is your job to immediately address it. It's a very different kind of stress, but stress nonetheless.

You can have patients with subarachnoid hemorrhages who are suddenly developing hydrocephalus, septic patients on four different drips to increase their blood pressure, patients with active GI bleeds profusely bleeding from their rectum, patients with impellas who cannot move a muscle, and patients with very emotional families surrounding everyone all the time. Oh, and the guy next door has basically been coding for the last two hours.

I will go over some time management tips specific to critical care and discuss my ideal timeline.

Critical care time management tips

1.   **Have a consistent routine.**

If you do this, you won't miss things. Rarely do things work perfectly, but you need to have a consistent, efficient, and comprehensive routine that you stick to when circumstances allow. Otherwise you could miss something important. Additionally, having a consistent routine can prevent you from getting behind early.

2.   **Stay ahead.**

Always have your charting done, even if you think you have nothing pressing going on. Things change quickly and severely in intensive care. You could suddenly get a coding admission and be in that room for hours, and if you didn't have your stable patient's assessment charted from two hours ago, you'll never remember it now. So if you're ahead on your meds but aren't caught up on charting, it is not the time to go grab coffee. Chart everything first, turn your patients, and make sure there is absolutely nothing left for you to do before you take a break.

3.   **Anticipate and prepare.**

Once you're in intensive care for a little while, you'll be able to predict how patients respond to certain things. For example, if I have a patient with a history of congestive heart failure who needs four units of fresh frozen plasma, I know I'm going to need some Lasix at some point; otherwise, Mr. Maddock is going to turn into Mr. Respiratory Distress. Additionally, if

I'm about to do a bedside tracheostomy placement, I know I'll need to have a bolus primed and ready to go. Typically, patients become hypotensive with the procedural meds administered. If you anticipate and prepare, you won't have to frantically grab supplies while your patient is decompensating. Every second counts.

4. Be meticulous.

Most nurses in intensive care have type-A personalities and are very meticulous and detailed. If you don't care about the details, you can miss something big, and it would be your fault. Meticulous nurses save lives because they know everything about their patient. And not only that, they care about the details. Say goodbye to being task-oriented—you are now big-picture oriented, and you won't be able to see and interpret the big picture if you don't know the details off the top of your head. Additionally, when things go downhill (because they can, quickly) you will know the important stuff off the top of your head for quick problem-solving in the midst of chaos.

5. Figure out what you think about death.

I know this is odd to say, but I highly recommend soul searching to figure out what you personally believe happens after a person dies, because you're going to see it. Frequently. It can be pretty heart-wrenching, and it can hit close to home. Make sure you have a good emotional support system so that when you have a really sad day, you can go talk to someone you trust and love. Nurses who don't have someone to talk to can become angry, sad, difficult to be around, and jaded. Moral distress is the number one cause of caregiver burnout. If you can't process death, it'll get to you eventually. Posttraumatic stress disorder (PTSD) in critical care nurses (and all other nurses) is real; please take care of your heart and soul.

6. Develop rapport with your physicians and other members of the health care team.

Things change very quickly in critical care. However, sometimes you just get a feeling about something and you need doctors who will listen to you, even when you don't have something concrete to tell them. I also suggest taking time to get to know your respiratory therapists. In intensive care, you will be working closely with them, so it's important to have a good relationship. Take the time to get to know them and develop a trusting relationship with the team you'll be working with frequently. It will pay off not only for you and the rest of the team, but for your patients as well.

7. **Don't trust the previous nurse.**

Verify everything yourself. "But I heard in report that…" is not an excuse. You need to verify your orders yourself. Just because the previous nurse said their blood pressure limits were 180–220 doesn't mean they are unless you physically see it in the chart. Rarely is this intentional or negligent. People miss things, transpose numbers, jumble data. When dealing with so many details, they can be mixed up easily. So read the physician's notes, look at CT scans, pull up the labs, and look at the medication list.

8. **Have a systematic way of reviewing the chart and documenting.**

In critical care, you are diving deep into the chart, looking closely at lab values, various diagnostics, medications that are currently being administered and medications that were previously administered in various locations, assessment findings, and so forth. Whenever you are giving and receiving report, go through it the same way every time so you know you're not missing something. Whenever you sit down to chart, do so in a systematic way. I liked to chart the patient's vitals and pain first, then the assessment, intake and output, lines, drains, and airways, followed by restraints and any additional documentation flow sheets that were applicable. It doesn't matter if your routine is different, just as long as you have one.

9. **Have a systematic way of reviewing and assessing your patient.**

With so many things attached to the patient, it's helpful to have a routine in place whenever you walk in to check them out. Before I even touched the patient, I would look at the monitor to ensure the alarm limits reflected the current order. I would make sure the head-of-bed height was appropriate, then level and zero my lines. I'd double-check each pump, all the tubing, and each of the bags to see if I needed to grab another one. If the ventilator was connected or the patient was on oxygen, I would verify that the machine was situated the way it needed to be. Then I would look at the patient head to toe. After that, I'd grab and administer my medications and finally, I would chart.

Critical care timeline

As you can imagine, the way you approach your day in critical care is very different than the way you approach your day on another unit. Here is my general timeline after I get report on my two patients. Typically, one patient is sicker than the other.

After or during report, I double-check my active orders while I'm looking at my lines, IV bags, and pump. I make sure I've got enough in all of the bags to get to my next med pass, verify that the pumps accurately reflect the med being administered, and take note if I need to change any tubing during the shift.

I make sure my monitor matches my ordered parameters (for example, if my order is to keep their systolic blood pressure between 120 and 150, I make sure the monitor is set appropriately). I check if there's anything I have to do (meds, labs, scans, etc.) at 0800. I print and interpret my telemetry strips.

I plan to go see my sicker patient first. I get any 0800 meds and supplies, complete my assessment, turn, give meds and oral care, and talk to them about the plan for the day. If time allows, I immediately chart my assessment at the bedside.

I again check all lines and tubes to insure that everything is up-to-date and where it needs to be. I also level and zero lines at this time.

Then, I go grab any 0800 and 0900 meds and supplies for my second (less sick) patient. I complete the same process as above with this patient and immediately chart what I've done. I usually end up administering medications last because it's barely 0800 by this time, and I have to wait until then to give the 0900 meds. Sometimes I even chart my entire assessment first and then go back to administer meds.

Then I head back into my first patient's room with their 0900 meds. If they are a q2h neuro check (meaning a full neurological assessment needs to be completed and documented every two hours), I complete and chart it at this time.

If my second patient is also a q2h neuro check, I complete and document that check.

Typically, if no one decompensates or needs to travel, and if no doctors round, I'm caught up by 0930.

This is an ideal timeline. However, it doesn't happen too often like that. Sometimes you come in and someone is not doing well at all, so they absorb your time and attention for a while. But it's important to establish your "this is what I do every day when time allows" routine.

Holistic care and intuition

In talking about so many tasks, it's hard not to get inundated by them. I'd like to tell you a story about another important aspect of providing nursing care in the midst of all these tasks. Being able to take the emotional temperature of the room is important. Rarely do people clearly communicate their emotional needs; most time they must be observed. This ability to observe is how we, as nurses, emotionally care for our patients.

I'd like to share with you a scenario in which I had to take some time and reflect on the emotional climate, which ultimately changed how I approached providing care for a patient and their loved one.

It was a pretty typical neuro ICU kind of day. I had two patients in the rooms right next to each other. They both were pretty sick but in very different ways.

One man was an alcoholic who had fallen and had a large subdural hematoma, as well as seizures. He had surgery to evacuate the hematoma. He did not have a breathing tube or majorly invasive lines and tubes, but he was still one sick pup. He was detoxing from alcohol, so he was agitated and difficult to control. Nonetheless, he was my patient, and I was determined to take good care of him. His family wasn't there much; I'm not sure if that was because they couldn't handle the ICU environment or because they simply didn't want to be there.

My other patient was another typical neuro ICU patient: a woman on a blood thinner who had fallen and hit her head. She had a traumatic subarachnoid hemorrhage, an intracerebral hemorrhage, and an intraventricular hemorrhage. Another sick pup. She had a breathing tube and was not doing a whole lot neurologically.

Her family was a little different than the family of my first patient. They never left her bedside. They would take turns going to the bathroom so the patient was never alone. They went through box after box of tissues, their faces constantly wet with tears. Every beep and alarm sent them into their own hypertensive crisis.

I could immediately tell that this family needed support. They needed my presence. They needed to trust me with their mom and wife. The emotional climate was cold, untrusting, and anxious.

Once I keyed into this, I explained every single thing before I did it, no matter how insignificant. I made sure they had ample tissues. I asked them how they were doing emotionally with a reassuring pat on the back. I told them I was sorry. I stayed present in those moments and really listened to them. While their loved one probably couldn't comprehend what I said to her, I made sure to explain everything to the patient before I did it. That meant more to them than I realized.

While it did take some time, it paid off in the long run. Once they felt supported and trusted me with her, they relaxed. They unclenched. They felt safe. They stopped asking so many questions and overreacting to every alarm.

Halfway through the day, her husband came up to me as I was about to give her yet another dose of Nimotop. He stopped me and said, "Now, I know I'm not supposed to know anything about other patients. But I walk by next door every time I go to the bathroom. I've seen how little his family is there. I've seen how rambunctious he can get. But more importantly, I've seen how well you take care of him when his family isn't there. I've seen you support him, even though he doesn't know what the heck is going on. I've seen how well you've taken care of my wife, myself, and my kids as we're going through this nightmare.

"That's why right now I'm going to go home for the first time in four days to shower," he said as he started to cry. "I trust you with her. I know you're going to take just as good care of my wife as you have your other patient when his family isn't around. I will be back before your shift is over, but I just wanted you to know that." He then gave me one of those awkward, manly "thank you" pats on the back.

I gave him a pat back, and we just stood there in silence for a few moments, gazing at his wife. I then hugged him and thanked him for what he said and for allowing me to take part in caring for his family.

I'll never forget that moment.

I didn't say anything profound all day. I didn't put together the pieces of some intricate clinical picture or call the doctor and suggest the perfect thing to improve the outcome. I didn't manage my time perfectly. I'm pretty sure at least one of my doses of Nimotop was late.

Letting go of trying to fix their emotional pain, assessing their needs, and just being there was the best I could do for them that day. If I had been put in that situation at the beginning of my career, I would have busted my butt charting perfectly, getting meds on time, and constantly trying to think of the perfect thing to say to them because I thought that was all that mattered. I would have been emotionally absent trying to fix that situation, ultimately feeling like a failure because *there is no perfect thing to say*. Sometimes patients and their loved ones just need a little extra explanation and reassurance. Sometimes they need you to prove to them that you know what you're doing and that their loved one is as important to you as they are to them. Sometimes they just need you to be emotionally present and acknowledge the difficulty of the situation.

Loved ones can try to put on a brave face for the patient because they don't want them to know they are scared. The same is true for patients. Acknowledging the situation lets them know that it is okay to break down and cry. It is okay for them to experience those emotions—they don't have to be brave for their nurse. Sometimes the best emotional support you can provide a person is just giving them permission to experience their emotions in a nonjudgmental atmosphere.

This builds trust.
This builds confidence.
This is nursing care.

Chapter 8

Dealing with Tough Patients and Loved Ones

While most of the time your patients are compliant and want to do whatever they can to get home, not all are as agreeable or motivated. I was grossly unprepared to deal with mean, demeaning, rude, or frustrating patients and their loved ones. I was also grossly unprepared to deal with difficult patients who, because of their medical conditions, were uncooperative.

Mean and demeaning patients bring my Nurse Face out. If you've been a nurse for more than twelve minutes, you know that some people are, well, jerks. Just like life outside of the hospital environment, some people are just not nice people.

Remember, there are many reasons why patients are difficult. They could have just received a life-altering diagnosis. They could be painfully frustrated by the lack of support from their family. They might normally use alcohol or smoking to deal with stress and right now they can't use their normal coping mechanism. They could also have underlying mental health issues that are impairing their judgment or perception of reality. There are a lot of very real and understandable variables that could impede their ability to receive care.

I want to walk through some very important things you need to know when you suddenly find yourself being spoken to in a rude way, making you feel disrespected or demeaned.

First Things First: You Deserve Respect

It's essential to understand that even though someone is ill or going through something really tough, this is not an excuse to be rude, demeaning, demanding, or inappropriate. You deserve respect. And sometimes when people are being rude as an unhealthy way of dealing with their situation, you need to *command* respect from them. There is absolutely no excuse or reason to treat you poorly. You do *not* deserve it.

Sometimes when people are going through something tough they lash out at those who are helping them. It can be a natural way for them to deal with something that's totally out of their control. While that may be how they're instinctively dealing with something, it does not make it okay. They may just need a little firm, but respectful, reminder that there are better ways to deal with difficult situations.

At the beginning of my career, I didn't know how much grace to extend to people who were a little rude here and there, or said something inappropriate, but at this point, I feel very confident with knowing where to draw the line. Whenever I start to personally feel uncomfortable or start to avoid going into the room, that's the line.

Three Practical Steps to Handling This

I have a few key steps to dealing with this situation.

> **Step 1.** Respond.
> **Step 2.** Don't treat them differently after.
> **Step 3.** Don't take it personally and carry it with you throughout the shift.

Naturally, you must respond in the situation in the moment first. In the box on the next page are some of my go-to responses.

I use one, a combination of two, or all four. This typically shuts this disrespect down quickly. You usually don't need to elaborate anymore because this snaps them out of their rudeness. I typically find that people get so wrapped up in their own experience, needs, and immediate priorities that they don't realize how ridiculous they're being. They usually profusely apologize.

Go-To Responses

You must respond with confidence, a stern, yet calm voice, and a serious face.

"That is inappropriate."

"You will not speak to me in that manner."

"Do not curse at me."

"As your nurse, I am here to help you, not be disrespected."

You're basically saying to the patient: "Hey, don't treat me like that. It's understandable that you're frustrated with everything, but you're taking it out on me. It's okay if that was your instinct, but you need to know that it's not okay to talk to me like that and we've gotta change how you're dealing with this. I'm still going to take really good care of you, even though we had this little bump in the road. Being sick sucks. I get it. And if you want to talk about it, I'm here."

Stopping the behavior is step one. Step two is how you treat them the rest of your shift. You must still provide great care. You dropped the "you must respect me" bomb, but you cannot shun them or their loved ones for the rest of the shift. Do not avoid interactions; still care for them as you would care for anyone else. I typically find that people are nicer and more considerate after we have this heart to heart.

However, if they do not respond by apologizing and changing their behavior, you must be consistent. Continually call out the inappropriate behavior, not the person (a tip from my husband, the counselor). If it persists, this may turn into a situation in which security or your manager needs to be pulled into the conversation. You should *never* feel unsafe or uncomfortable while you're providing nursing care. Never.

Finally, step three of this situation is to not take it personally. It can be hard to do this sometimes, but it is essential. I find it helpful to kind of step outside of the situation in my mind and remind myself that this person is going through a lot and needs a reminder (some more forceful than others) of how to act, and that this is their way dealing with the world, not mine. Regardless of how they treat me, I know and hold to the facts: that I am doing the best I can to care for them and that I'm a wonderful, caring person. They can say whatever horrible things they can think of, but it will not change how I feel about myself. Hold strong to that truth and don't let a patient, their family member, or anyone else take that from you. Guard your heart and mind when things get volatile.

Confused and mean

Sometimes you'll have patients who are pretty difficult to deal with because of a disease process that makes them not of sound mind. You need to deal with this differently. Speaking as a neuro ICU nurse, I've dealt with this many times.

Hopefully, if they're suffering from acute confusion, you're working with the health care team to identify and treat the cause. However, there are many patients who are confused at baseline. Take your normally slightly confused patient, put them in a hospital, and on top of that add in being sick—now it's a whole new ballgame.

In these situations, it's essential to decide which battles are worth fighting. For example, if my super irritated patient detoxing from alcohol is flipping out about taking medications, I'm not going to spend twenty minutes convincing him to take his scheduled stool softener. The stool softener is not a priority anymore. His blood pressure medications and Ativan* are.

I'm going to crush those, throw it in some applesauce, and try to get him to take that one bite for me. If I think it's going to be a problem or feel unsafe, I'll call my buds in security to stand right next to me while he takes them. When the doctor rounds, I'll make sure to touch base with them about the challenges I'm having with medication administration.

Sometimes, you'll have someone whose confusion is escalating and who is not responding to your reasoning. I find that it can be helpful to call security *before* they get too heated. This person may need to see someone in a uniform. Even through the fog of confusion, a security guard in a uniform can calm people down. Usually the act of requesting security communicates the seriousness of the situation, even to some confused patients. However, I often still talk with security and ask them to explain to the patient how to treat the staff.

(Also, shout-out to security officers. I sincerely appreciate you and the support you provide to the nursing staff. It means a lot to me and I feel very safe because of you.)

---

* **Nursepedia Definition:** *Ativan* is typically given to patients withdrawing from alcohol to combat the symptoms, which can include seizures, delirium tremens (DTs), and agitation.

I hope this helps you as you have those tough patients. I remember feeling so bad and beat down when patients were mean and treated me like the lowest of the low. But once I got my mind around the situation, I felt empowered. I began to feel armed to deal with these situations and therefore didn't try to avoid them. I now take them on immediately and address the behavior. It makes the shift go much better, and typically the patient and I have a much deeper, trusting relationship because they know I'll call them out when they're being ridiculous and still support them.

Avoid the Power Struggle

Do not get into a power struggle for the benefit of your ego. Some nurses will get quite bent out of shape when a patient does not do as they're instructed. Getting mad about noncompliance is worthless; it will just stress you out and make it more difficult to provide care. You cannot try to force these patients to participate. Pick the really important things and try to figure out how you can increase compliance in these areas. I have had one patient during my career refuse most nursing care. I had a few conversations with him about what refusing vital signs and assessments meant. He verbalized that he understood and was of sound mind, so I documented thoroughly and went about my shift. I could not physically force him to do anything and therefore could only do my part of educating him on the implications of his actions and documenting this appropriately.

Tips for Dealing with Specific Demeanors (No, not Dementors…Demeanors)

As I mentioned before, people can be difficult, in their right mind or not, in different ways. Here are some tips on how I go about dealing with different situations.

Grouchy, grumpy, or mad about doing anything

Befriend them, joke with them, figure out something they like or care about and bring it up a few times. Be on their side. Don't push too much conversation or linger too long. Be casual and treat them like an average Joe. Then when you need them to do something, present the task as a favor.

Belligerent or combative

You must have a strong and confident presence with these patients. Keep in mind: Strong and confident is different than loud and demanding.

Immediately stop them if they curse at you and calmly inform them that they will not speak to you in that manner. Cursing gets people hyped up and it's good to stop that in its tracks.

I never hesitate to call security if someone is combative and difficult to physically control. Know how to tie restraints, how to push antipsychotics safely (you can't just slam them in), and the number for security. You must ensure you have the appropriate orders for both chemical and physical restraints. Unfortunately, both are necessary sometimes. Once you deal with a few of these situations, you'll know what to do, and you'll become more confident each time.

I think some people are hesitant to call security or request support because they don't want to be an alarmist or overly react to a situation. Honestly, many of us are hesitant to act or request support out of fear of judgment of others.

Regardless, please do not work under the assumption that because you're a nurse, you should just take it in stride and should only stop the behavior when it's really bad. You have the right to feel comfortable and safe at work, so when you begin to not feel comfortable and safe, it's time to bring in reinforcements. I've spoken with many individuals on this topic, and one PA said to me that whenever he told a nurse to call security when he observed unsafe or inappropriate behavior, the nurse seemed to have a sense of relief. It's helpful if someone outside of the situation can say, "This has escalated and needs to stop." It provides quite a bit of support to the nurse who is experiencing the behavior and presents a team mentality.

I remember when I was shadowing a nurse who was caring for a young traumatic brain injury patient during my nurse residency program. He was pretty intact neurologically, but intermittently, he'd just be a little dazed and off.

We were sitting at the nurse's station looking at another patient's chart when we heard him start screaming angrily. The nurse I was shadowing immediately popped up out of her chair and headed to his room. I was a bit nervous but followed her lead.

Apparently, he had spilled some water or juice on his lap, and it set him off. He was screaming and cursing loudly. He wasn't just screaming at himself, he was screaming at the nurse as well in a very explicit manner.

He said about two curse words in this tone before she said, "Stop! I am your nurse, and I am here to take care of you. You will *not* speak to me like that. There are other patients on this unit, and you are disturbing them by screaming. This is not appropriate."

This snapped him out of it immediately. He profusely apologized. Due to his injury, his moods and emotions were all over the place, and this was one of the first times he'd had an angry outburst. It was empowering to see that her immediate reaction was to not tolerate the behavior, even though it was related to his disease process.

If I had been alone in that situation at that point in my career, I don't know what I would have done. I probably would have left the room immediately to get a new sheet, not stopping the behavior. I just didn't feel empowered at that point to stand up for myself like that. I do now and am glad I was able to observe that so early on in my career.

Demeaning

The first thing to remember about patients who are demeaning is the behavior may not be about you. They could be mad about something else, be it their disease process or another aspect in their life. When someone speaks to me in a demeaning manner, I reply in a very matter-of-fact tone, "I am here to care for you today, it is not appropriate to speak to me in that manner." Most of the time, that defuses the tension, and they feel bad for taking their anger out on their nurse and apologize.

If possible, I like to break down the mean wall and ask them about their lives. This usually softens their demeanor. However, not everyone responds to this method, and when that happens, I keep my interactions short and intentional. I extend a little grace, but I do not offer so much that I'm continually being disrespected.

In my entire career, I believe I have experienced only two patients who were truly mean or rude people.

Way too talkative or avoiding doing things

Some people are really great at manipulating other people, either by being extremely chatty and talking their way out of important aspects of their care, or just completely avoiding treatment. Some will keep putting things off all shift until it's too late, or every time you try to get them to eat, they just talk your ear off.

My tip is to engage in conversation with them, but know when to stop conversation and have them refocus on the task at hand. I always pretend it's the doctor's fault and say something like: "The doctor insists you get out of bed three times today, no excuses. Let's get the first one out of the way now."

(Thanks, docs!) Again, engage in conversation but frequently redirect conversation to the task at hand.

When it's the family making things challenging

In addition to patients being difficult to care for, occasionally we have to deal with families and loved ones who are as well. Generally speaking, most loved ones and families care deeply for the patient and want only the best for them. However, they're stressed to the max, feel very helpless, and are way out of their comfort zone. It's completely understandable that they aren't acting as they normally would.

It is important to remember that most patients and loved ones are not familiar with the medical system. They don't know when to be concerned, therefore everything is concerning. You and the physicians are all speaking a totally different language. They just met you and the physicians, so they don't trust you yet. And they don't live in this medical world every day like you do. Remember to have some extra grace and understanding. Even if they come off rude, demeaning, frustrated, or passive aggressive, usually at the bottom of all of that is *fear*.

Dealing with it throughout the shift

First of all, when you hear in report that the family is difficult, you need to consciously step up your patience game. You'll need more patience today than you would normally. All of your interactions are going to have to be intentional, and you're going to have to try harder with them than your other patients and families, because they need it. Everything you do or don't do, they'll watch and analyze. Every time you walk into that room, walk in with confidence, and have intentional conversations.

What I mean by intentional is that you have purpose behind everything you say to them. You're not just flippantly chitchatting; you mean business. Compassionate and caring business.

Below is how I have intentional conversations. It was a little difficult and awkward at first, but now it's like clockwork and I don't think about it anymore.

I always enter the room and introduce myself to my patient first. I tell them my name, shake their hand, and inform them that I'll be their nurse all day. I don't know why, but this simple gesture can mean a lot to someone. It tells them that they are not just another patient to me; they are a person

I'm happy to be meeting for the first time. During my introduction, I speak directly to the patient first (if they are conscious). Everything is about the patient. Family or no family, this person still needs your care, and they should be the center of everything you do.

During this time, I will occasionally look at whoever else is there. When I'm done with that, I ask the patient, "So who is this you've got here with you today?" I shake their hand(s) as well and introduce myself to them after I've spoken with the patient directly. It establishes a professional tone.

If the loved one is already mad, hopefully that defuses their frustration. Maybe they hated the nurse last night, and the doctor was short with them yesterday. Maybe no one has really explained to them what's going on, and they feel completely out of the loop. There are a million reasons people are rude, overbearing, mean, condescending, and so on. However, let them know through your actions and conversation that you are here now. It is a new day, and you are a new nurse to the situation, and you are going to have a fantastic day.

You want them to feel safe and know that you're going to take good care of their loved one. Making your presence and authority known initially tends to make them feel better about leaving their loved one in your care. It reassures them. You want them to trust you. The more they trust you, the more freedom they'll give you to care for the patient.

When you have that initial conversation at the beginning of your shift, let them know what the deal is for the day. Discuss things like general goals for the shift, when you can loosely predict the doctor will be around, when and what meds will be given, and so forth.

It's common for loved ones to feel an "us versus them" mentality when someone is hospitalized, especially if the health care team failed to meet their expectations, or the support system is very overwhelmed and confused. Additionally, many people just generally struggle with trust. Trusting people right away is a challenge for most, and suddenly their loved one is hospitalized and at the complete mercy of a bunch of strangers. It's helpful to consistently speak from a "we're on the same team" mentality. Proactive education, explaining things before they happen, and providing predictability really facilitates this mindset.

Predictability is something that reassures even the most scared family members, more than anything else. Remember this as you're interacting with them. Even if you think you're being redundant, go over the plan again. You are in charge and it enhances your professionalism and their trust in you. If you know what you're doing and they can sense that, it makes them unclench a bit. You don't just want the patient to feel safe, you want the loved ones to feel this way as well.

Sometimes patients are also worried about their loved ones. Loved ones are worrying about the patient, the patient is worrying about the loved ones, and everyone is just one big ball of stress. Calm, caring confidence from you will make all the difference to every single one of them.

Also, I try to keep things light, when appropriate, because patients and loved ones really appreciate that. Typically, the patient is in the hospital for something sad, serious, or scary, so if you can make them laugh or talk about something not illness related, they light up. If their family member sees them smile, that speaks much louder than getting their meds right on time.

When the family goes too far

A frustrating family member throughout the shift is one thing, but what if they yell at you? Or what if they curse at you? Or what if they start scream-crying at you? All of those have happened to me before. I've been screamed at, called explicit names, and had to call security when family members became hostile.

I handle these situations similarly to how I handle it when a patient speaks to me like that. Just remember people are under immense duress and many don't have a good way to cope with it. Give it very little power in your heart and mind. Remember, do not take it personally.

A suggestion for what to say to family members like this would be:

> *I understand that it was really frustrating to hear the doctor say what she said. I know you had a lot of hope that your family member would walk out of here, and she just told you he wouldn't. Keep in mind that we're all on the same team. We're here to support you both through this. I'm really sorry you're going through this. I'm here for you. We want to be open and honest with you about what's going on, even if it's bad news. We don't want you to be in the dark.*

These "it just got real" conversations never happen at the end of your shift. They're always two hours in when you have ten more hours to deal with the family. Maintain your when you have additional interactions throughout the day.

An occasional joke goes a long way. Don't shun that person the rest of the day. It just creates more stress for you, makes caring for the patient more difficult, and is honestly kind of mean and immature on your part if that's how you choose to deal with these situations. Hook your patient up with some ice cream, a warm blanket, or something like that. If they know you're still going to take care of their loved one, they usually calm down eventually.

The wife I'll never forget

I'll always remember one family that would have been considered a difficult family but will always be near and dear to my heart.

The husband was diagnosed with colon cancer a few years prior, received treatment, and was in remission for a while. Well, he started to get confused at home and they brought him in and found out the cancer had spread to his brain. He was on vasoactive medications, tube feeding, and on and off the ventilator. One day he could readily wiggle his toes, the next he couldn't follow any commands.

Every time the monitor beeped, she panicked. Every time he made even the slightest of movements, she rejoiced. It was quite the emotional rollercoaster ride that ended up lasting weeks and weeks.

Rarely could the staff do anything right. Rarely did we get in the room fast enough. Rarely was she pleased with us. It took me a few weeks to realize that she wasn't upset with us; she was upset with the situation.

After being in the thick of it for weeks, many of us just couldn't emotionally take it anymore. Out of self-preservation, we'd switch off who cared for him.

Whenever a physician would come in, she'd focus solely on anything positive they might say, no matter how insignificant. If his white blood cell count went from fourteen to ten, it was a massive victory despite the fact that he was practically comatose. It started to take the focus away from the big picture of it all: He was dying. However, no matter how many physicians came in and told her the same thing, she was still full speed ahead. Palliative care or hospice was not an option. Not doing absolutely everything every single day was entirely neglectful in her eyes.

Eventually, a few physicians had a family meeting with her and the patient's siblings and his adult child, and it finally got through to her that absolutely everything had been done to save her husband. Despite this, he was deteriorating and would continue to do so. She reluctantly agreed to transfer to hospice.

Two other nurses from my unit, a physician, a nurse practitioner, and I, all who were closely involved during their entire stay, went and visited them. He was still in pain, but he finally looked comfortable, with fewer lines and tubes, and in a much cozier environment. It was a relief to see that he was going to be able to pass peacefully and didn't have to fight any longer.

I was able to tell the family some things that I couldn't tell them before because I was so frustrated that he was on our unit for so long. I was able to tell her that I was glad he had a wife who loved him so dearly and that he clearly loved her deeply. She told me some stories about him and just seemed softer in her interactions. I think it meant a lot to her that we came down to see them that day and offer our condolences and gratitude for allowing us to participate in his care.

While he was on our unit, I was frustrated and upset. I was so mad at the wife and couldn't comprehend her decisions. I hated when I came into work after a few days off and saw him still in our unit, still getting poked, getting test after test.

But when I went down there to offer my condolences to them, all of that went away. The cloud of frustration lifted when I finally was able to empathize. I don't know exactly how I would act if my husband and best friend was lying in an intensive care unit, slightly responsive some days and comatose the rest, but I would definitely want to push for every possible option that might miraculously breathe life into him again, so I could have my best friend back. I probably would stop at nothing to ensure that no stone was left unturned before I relinquished and said, "Enough. Let him go home. I'll meet him there."

Chapter 9

The Code Blues

To start out my chapter on code blues, I'd like to share with you my first code blue.

My First Code Blue

I was a few weeks out of orientation and working the night shift on a cardio-vascular and thoracic surgery step-down unit. The three other nurses and I had finished our med passes and assessments and were just sitting down to get our documentation done. The techs were going around room to room to do vitals. All was well in our world.

One of the telemetry alarms started going off, a usual occurrence on our floor.

I looked up from my computer to see the patient's heart rate flashing in red. It was 36.

"Not too bad, I've seen worse," I thought. "She's probably really asleep and normally drops this low. I'll go check on her for my coworker because she's with another patient." I got up and walked to her room across from the nurse's station.

I walked in the dark room. "Ma'am... Ma'am..." I said as I walked closer to her. A coworker was behind me and yelled, *"She's not breathing call the code!"*

As I rushed to the head of the patient's bed, I thought, "Man, how did she see that? It's so dark in here. I should have noticed that immediately."

Just before the code was called overhead to summon the troops, I heard our emergency red telephone ring at the desk. It was the telemetry monitors on another floor, calling to tell us the patient had flipped into a deadly heart rhythm.

I frantically searched for the CPR lever that's on all hospital beds and couldn't find it. I gave up and tried to get her head positioned to put the bag-valve mask on her face. I didn't know what I was doing. I guessed that was the next best thing to do. I was in that weird mental state of knowing I needed to act incredibly fast but feeling clueless about what to do.

Luckily the most experienced nurse had her head together. I felt like an idiot. She found and pulled the CPR lever immediately. She directed the tech to start chest compressions while she slapped the defibrillator pads on the patient. The tech started compressions.

"She needs to push harder, lower, and faster," I thought. "But what do I know? I've never done this before. The experienced nurse hasn't said anything, so she must be doing okay. I hope."

I heard the code cart coming down the hall. Those things are always so loud.

The woman had had open-heart surgery the week before. The large incision down the middle of her chest was still stapled together and the staples were soon soaked with blood from the new damage.

Respiratory therapy arrived and took over my fumbling attempts to clear her airway. I took over CPR. I didn't even put gloves on; I just started compressions. For some reason, I didn't even think about it. All I could think about was minimizing the time between compressions, so I pushed harder, lower, and faster. No one said anything.

The the ICU nurses and ED nurses)and in-house hospitalist with his residents showed up. They took over. I stepped back and watched, feeling helpless for this poor woman who hadn't been on the brink of death four minutes ago.

They did the typical rounds of IV push meds to try to get her heart back in a normal rhythm. They stuck a breathing tube down her throat. The ICU and ER nurses showed me how to do real chest compressions. The hospitalist made the residents take turns. They got blood on the sleeves of their freshly pressed white coats.

In the midst of the controlled chaos, the house supervisor asked, "Has anyone called the family?"

The family. I forgot about the family.

"Not that we know, we're coding her!" yelled someone from the room. The house supervisor told the charge nurse to call the family and tell them to get here. Now.

I tried to help in any way that I could. I ran to get saline flushes and IV pumps, primed IV tubing, wrote things down but somehow felt like I didn't do a thing. I looked at the nurse pulling meds from the code cart seamlessly, the one pushing them in the patient's central line and calling the meds out with the time so the recorder knew what he was doing, and the one doing compressions so well that I could see it on the monitor.

"How do they know how to do this? And how do I not?" I thought.

Thirty-five minutes passed.

Nothing.

"We have been coding her for thirty-five minutes and have had no response," said the doctor. "We will attempt one more shock, and if that doesn't work, we will call it."

"Clear the patient," said the ICU nurse who was at the defibrillator. Everyone stepped back from the patient. "Shocking!" she said, as she pushed the blinking orange button.

The shock caused the patient's chest to momentarily jump up off of the bed. We all stared at the monitor in silence.

She had flatlined.

"Time of death: 2342," said the doctor as he took off his bloody gloves.

Everyone stopped what they were doing, threw away what was in their hands, and immediately left the room. The doctor signed what he needed to and left. The ICU and ER nurses did the same. One of my coworkers printed a telemetry strip of her flatline to put in the chart.

The nurse who was taking care of the patient was crying in the hallway. The family started walking down the hallway toward the nurse's station. We all looked at each other to see who was going to step up and tell them. The doctor was already gone and probably wasn't coming back. The daunting responsibility somehow fell on her. I think the family put the pieces together when they saw her crying.

Through her tears, the nurse told them she didn't make it.

You could hear a blunt needle drop. We all stood in silence as she delivered the news. I'd never seen anyone receive the news that their loved one had died. Out of respect, I tried not to watch, but I knew that I would be in her shoes one day, breaking the news to a family, trying to find the right words to say.

A few family members were pretty quiet and stoic. One was very angry and upset, and the rest were crying.

A few others and I went into the room to clean her up to make her presentable for the family. We cleaned up all of the blood that oozed out of the foot-long incision on her chest, closed her eyes by holding them down for thirty seconds, and discarded the remnants of the code. The trash cans were full of empty medication vials, syringes, wrappers, and bloody gloves.

After we gave them the all clear, the family members filed in and closed the door. Once they were all in the room, we all exhaled a little.

The house supervisor comforted the nurse who was in shock about what had happened in the last forty-five minutes. There was literally nothing she could have done differently. Unfortunately, that was one of the risks of the surgery the patient had undergone. It doesn't happen too often, but when it does, it reminds you that, no matter how advanced our medical technology gets, we're all still human. The nurse pulled it together and started charting; she had to call the coroner soon.

The house supervisor went in and asked the family members if they wanted an autopsy and which funeral home they wanted to go with. Once they said they didn't want an autopsy, we went in and took out all of her lines, tubes, and airway.

I went in and removed her breathing tube, central line, and urinary catheter.

I used surgical lube to wiggle her wedding band off of her cold, swollen finger to give to her family.

The family went in one more time to see her as they had always seen her, without the large breathing tube down her throat and her head cocked as far back as it could go. They left one by one with bloodshot eyes and heavy hearts in a complete daze.

I went back in with my tech, put her in a body bag, and placed a tag on her foot.

The funeral home was called. They'd be here in an hour to pick her up, after which the room would be cleaned and that nurse would be open for an admission.

Code Blues for Newbies

Seeing a cardiac or respiratory arrest for the first time is a pretty shocking event. It's hard to process when you see it the first few times. It's hard to quickly snap into "go mode" to do the emergency, life-saving tasks.

Here are some things for you to do in a code situation when you don't know what to do.

As you may know, the BLS and ACLS* policies have been updated to say that compressions are the number-one priority. Compressions must be done before anyone does anything else. Someone needs to be on their chest, cracking their ribs. (Yes, if you feel their ribs breaking under your hands that means you're doing it right.)

The code cart has a backboard that breaks off and needs to be placed under the patient. If I hear a code and am running down the hall next to someone with the cart, I rip it off and bring it in with me, even if compressions aren't indicated yet. I get the backboard under the patient so compressions can start immediately when necessary.

If someone is taking care of compressions, the next thing to address is the airway. Every single hospital room should have a bag-valve mask connected to oxygen tubing at the head of the bed. Connect the mask to the oxygen valve on the wall and crank it all the way up. Tilt their head all the way back, seal the mask over their nose and mouth, and squeeze the bag to administer breaths.

The code cart should have portable suction. If the room doesn't already have suction set up, go ahead and turn that bad boy on. Suction is used to clear secretions from the patient's airway, which is essential during intubations or when someone has a compromised airway. Typically, respiratory therapy shows up very quickly and takes over for airway management. It is very helpful if you have this set up and started for them so they can just hop into your place.

---

* **Nursepedia Definition:** *BLS* (basic life support) nurses can provide CPR and *ACLS* (advanced cardiac life support) nurses can push meds per the ACLS algorithms without a physician.

In every single code, the defibrillator needs to be attached to the patient. Most code carts are set up so that you can unplug the defibrillator from the code cart and set it on the bed. The faster this is done, the better. Even if your patient is on telemetry, is in a respiratory arrest, and still has a pulse, get the defibrillator on. The pads will indicate where they need to be placed on the patient. Once the pads are on the patient, turn on the defibrillator and position it so that the physician can see the patient's rhythm from where they are standing.

All right, what else do we need? IV access. Make sure the patient has some sort of access; if not, start working on another IV. Hopefully, they already do, and one of your ACLS-certified nurses is pulling meds and drawing them up from the code cart while the other is pushing them.

If you get chest compressions started, get the bag-valve mask on the patient, have the defibrillator attached and on the bed, and have IV access, your code team will thank you. It's as if you're a basketball team that only ever runs one play, and the "code blue" being announced overhead is the call to get down the court to set up. The situation (where the defense is) will guide what your next steps are, but the interventions remain the same. Getting these things done for your team is the perfect setup.

Ideally, there are two people for compressions (one performing them and one ready to switch), three ACLS RNs (pushing meds, pulling them, and announcing the ACLS algorithm and times), an MD, an RN documenting, one runner, one to two respiratory therapists at the head of bed, and the primary nurse telling the doctor what happened. There shouldn't be more than that in the room. If you were doing something in that room and the code team arrived to take over, immediately exit the room.

Sometimes, things can get loud and chaotic in a code. Communication must be concise and clear. Sometimes people get a little frantic and yell or are not incredibly polite. Please try not to take anything personally from people in the midst of this intense situation.

Qualities of a Smoothly Run Code

1. It's quiet and calm. No one is shouting. People calmly ask questions and request supplies. No one speaks unless it is pertinent to the care that's being provided.
2. The only interruptions to CPR are during designated pulse checks after two-minute cycles and during shocks. (Yes, you need to keep doing compressions while the defibrillator is charging).

3. Someone is with the family. It can be easy to forget about them when a code is called; make sure someone is with them. If the family isn't already at the bedside, make sure someone is calling them.

4. Everyone moves efficiently. Every second counts.

5. Actions are documented and orders are entered in real time. Sometimes, this is only possible if you have experienced people at the computer or cart, because doing this during a code takes quite a bit of practice.

6. The patient's primary nurse tells the physician exactly, yet quickly, what's going on with the patient and what led up to the code, and stays nearby for any questions that may come up.

7. Someone is able to look things up quickly and efficiently in the patient's chart (labs, last chest x-ray, recent tests and procedures, etc.).

8. If it's a small room, someone takes out unnecessary items. If everyone who needs to be in the room is there and there's a huge recliner blocking the door, someone needs to move that recliner. Chances are, if the patient survives, the bed will be moved out of the room.

Also, keep in mind that a code on the floor runs differently than one in the ICU or ED. In the ICU or ED, rooms are usually bigger and the nurses, techs, and physicians are more familiar with codes. Patients typically have adequate IV access, they're already hooked up to telemetry, and ventilators and other advanced equipment are close by. Basically, ICU and ED codes tend to run more smoothly and be more efficient.

If you have the ability to go to a code in an ICU or ED just to watch, I highly encourage it. It's quite an experience to just observe. It's almost artistic and beautiful to see this team of people working together to save someone's life. The calm teamwork is amazing. The doctor asks for something and it's done immediately. The doctor asks a question and it gets answered. The things that just need to be done (applying and turning on the defibrillator, popping open the intubation kit, getting IV access, applying backboard, and priming a bolus) are already done or being done. No one has to ask.

Pro Nurse Tip: ICU and ED CNAs are awesome at CPR. If you want to learn how to do great chest compressions, go watch the CNAs in the ICU and ED. It is exhausting, but good chest compressions save people's lives. So, shout out to all of you CNAs out there. You make all the difference in the world.

My First Non–Code Blue Code Blue

"Code blue, room 672. Code blue, room 672. Code blue, room 672."

I heard it called overhead as I was charting my last assessment. My unit doesn't usually respond to code blues, but I was caught up and knew the other unit was a bit behind. I told my coworker I was going to respond to the code, gave her a short report, and ran off the unit to room 672.

I stepped off of the elevator onto the cancer floor. I saw the code cart and a crowd of people outside of the room.

I caught up with intensive care doctor and the rapid response nurse just before getting to the door. We exchanged silent greetings and walked into the room together.

In the bed was a frail man who couldn't have weighed more than 85 pounds. He was contracted, his head to the side, not breathing. Next to his bed stood his wife. She had white hair, a stained shirt, and was screaming, "Put the breathing machine on, what is wrong with you?" The patient's nurse ran into the room while holding back tears to explain the situation to the code team who was at the ready,.

"He's a DNR [do not resuscitate], everyone. I was in the room, with his wife, when he stopped breathing. I told her that he stopped breathing, and she demanded a CPAP [continuous positive airway pressure] machine to open up his airway. I told her that he's a DNR and asked if she was sure she wanted me to call a code and she said yes."

The patient's wife started screaming again through tears. She didn't understand that the machine wasn't going to make him breathe. She didn't understand what the CPAP machine did. All she knew was that her husband had stopped breathing and that people who had trouble breathing used a CPAP machine, so she assumed it would fix the problem.

It wouldn't.

As tears ran down her red face, she began to raise her voice again. The doctor started to calmly explain what we all already knew: The patient had died. And instead of holding his hand during his last breath, she was filled with anger and screaming at any- and everyone who walked into the room to attempt to help. Although at that point, the definition of "help" was somewhat unclear.

As the reality of the situation began to set in, the rapid response nurse and I stepped out and let the physician explain the situation privately.

About four minutes later, the physician walked out of the room. The wife stood in the corner of the room, defeated, crying, and in shock.

I came up to her, told her I was sorry, and asked if I could get her anything.

"Diet Coke would be nice. He just has regular in here and I can't drink that stuff."

"Sure, I'll get you that."

"Thanks," she said looking at the floor.

"Is there anyone I can call for you? A friend, family, a pastor?" I asked.

"No. There's no one. It's just me and him," she said, looking at her husband. "And now it's just me."

My heart sank to the floor. I had no clue what to say or do next, so I hugged her, and went to go get her diet Coke.

I walked into the hallway; everyone was standing at the nurse's station. I asked for the diet Coke and the CNA went to grab one. I could tell the patient's nurse, who had taken care of him for days, was pretty shaken up. Her eyes were red because she had been crying since the whole situation had started. "You did a good job, you did the right thing," I told her.

She smiled at me and quietly squeaked out a "thanks." Her eyes were filled with tears, but she was trying to hold them back. She had six other patients she needed to care for. Mid–med pass on a busy oncology unit at 0915 was not the time to get emotional. I'm sure she was already forty-five minutes behind at that point. My heart ached for her.

The CNA returned with the only thing I could offer the patient's wife, that darn diet Coke. I thanked her and headed back to the room.

As I was walking back in, the patient's oncologist walked into the room. The rapid response nurse was still in the room, asking her how long they'd been married and trying to offer some support and presence. After she answered, an awkward and painful silence filled the room. The physician, the rapid response nurse, and I had no idea what to say.

The rapid response nurse and I straightened the patient up in bed, pulled his covers back over him, and made him look as peaceful and comfortable as possible. Even if there had been chaos around him, he died quickly and without pain, something that seems like a rare occurrence in the hospital.

We all left the room to give her some privacy with her husband. The rapid response nurse stayed to do some paperwork. The oncologist was already in the next patient's room, carrying on with his rounding. The physician who originally talked to the wife was long gone. I slowly headed back to my unit.

Comfort Care Conversations

Not everyone in the hospital who dies goes through a code. Many people have predictable (or somewhat predictable) deaths. For every code I've gone to, I've sat through ten comfort care* conversations. Many times we realize a patient is going to die and need to sit down to talk to the patient and family about how we will proceed.

Sometimes in the hospital, it becomes apparent that if we continue providing life support or other aspects of treatment, we will only be prolonging the inevitable without providing any improved quality of life. You'd think that it would be painfully obvious when someone's health gets to that point, but it's not. Sometimes people are wide awake and completely interactive but know they don't want this breathing tube down their throat anymore.

Many times, as the nurse, you are the first person to bring up the need for a conversation about end-of-life decision-making, as you're the person who is with the patient all day. The physicians are great at picking up on patients whose clinical picture is very ominous, but it's the nurses who really notice the ones who may look okay on paper but, looking at the big picture, aren't doing so great.

Ideally, the doctor brings this up to the patient or family when it's clinically evident that nothing else can be done. When you know this conversation is about to happen, it's really important that you be in the room. It's tough, but you should be there. You're with them all day; your presence will be (or should be) comforting because they see you more than the doctor.

Sometimes we need to take the palliative care step before hospice or a comfort care measure. Palliative care is different than hospice, as you don't have to be dying to receive palliative care. Palliative care basically prevents suffering and relieves pain. You can be a twenty-five-year-old military veteran with an amputation and receive palliative care.

---

* **Nursepedia Definition:** *Comfort care* means that the goal of care is now to make the patient comfortable as they pass, rather than achieve a full recovery.

Palliative care is a wonderful thing. Nurses love it. Some physicians take more convincing. The mention of palliative care can make doctors cringe, especially surgeons. I think that when we mention palliative care, they think we're just giving up. Many physicians feel that they went into medicine to fix problems and to make people better. So admitting that we've gone as far as we can in one or multiple areas and need to refocus our goals can feel like failure to them. Regardless of how difficult it may be for a member of the health care team, we always need to advocate for what is best for the patient.

One of the great things about a palliative care team is they get everyone on the same page. They are great at painting a complete and consistent picture of the prognosis after getting direction from the physicians who have already been taking care of the patient.

Also, when a physician decides to consult palliative care or hospice, make sure the physician tells the family what they're doing. Someone could be set off if, without warning, a palliative care doctor or hospice nurse practitioner comes in and talks to them I've been there. I've seen it happen. I tried to smooth it over, but ultimately the physician lost all trust, credibility, and respect from a family going through something terrible. Make sure the doctor talks to the family about this, no matter how uncomfortable it may be.

While these conversations are not easy, I find nurses feel more comfortable in that uncomfortable space than many physicians. Take that opportunity to go support the physician delivering the news, help them communicate with the family, or be the emotional support to the family while the physician is providing the technical clinical information.

Keep in mind, certain religions do not believe at all in hospice or palliative care. I've had a few devout Muslim patients who prioritized the quantity of life over the quality. They fought for every single day that their loved one had on this earth, even if the patient was in pain and suffering. I had to keep their beliefs ahead of my own personal opinions. While the option for palliative and hospice care should still be presented, be aware that the patient and family may not respond positively, which is okay; our opinions don't really matter if that's what the patient would want.

A lot of times, families will think that taking the comfort care step means we have lost all hope, but what hope looks like changes when you walk through life and death. When they were admitted, the hope was that they'd go home. When they had the huge stroke, the hope was that they wouldn't need a feeding tube. When they became unresponsive, the hope was that they would regain consciousness. And when nothing could be done to get the patient home, functioning, and off a ventilator and multiple vasoactive drips, the hope became that they could die comfortably.

Your presence and attitude

Your tone should change a little bit after the goals of care have shifted from recovery to comfort. Focus on being more comforting, supportive, and reassuring rather than motivating and gung-ho with high spirits. These patients (if they're awake) and families are very emotional, understandably so. Try not to act differently if they cry. Ask if you can hug them.

Hugging an emotional family member was a bit odd for me at first, but once I watched a nurse I really looked up to hug a crying wife, I felt reassured that it was okay. That wife hugged her and cried so hard, and man, she really needed to. And she was so thankful that the nurse hugged her first.

What to say when you don't know what to say

A lot of times we're at a loss for words when dealing with these patients and families. We just don't know how to talk to them all of a sudden. That's okay; it's not a comfortable place to be, but we still need to be there for them. Sitting in silence with them is okay.

Something I have learned that goes a long way is just acknowledging what's going on, saying something like, "Mr. Smith, I just want you to know that I'm really sorry that you're going through this."

That says, "I'm here with you, I acknowledge this sucks, but we're going to walk through this and I'll be here to support you today." It can be a small amount of reassurance during a really rough time.

You're not going to make them feel better or take their pain away; you just need to be comforting and supportive. Support their decisions, empower them, and tell them that their loved one is lucky to have them there. I also have told families that, although this is a terrible situation, I have seen patients pass with no one at their side and that I think it's wonderful that so many people clearly love this person.

More than anything, these families want you to empathize with them. They do not want sympathy from you. They don't want you looking down on them, patting them on the back telling them everything will be okay. They want you to sit next to them and connect with them. Nothing you say will fix what's happening. Let go of that desire (much easier said than done, I know). Be content and comfortable sitting next to them while they cry. Connect with them. An "I'm so sorry you're going through this" goes a long way. Once you do it a few times, you'll get better, but it never gets easy.

You may also get a lot of "Why would [my deity] allow this?" and "Why is [my deity] taking them away from me?" questions. Everyone's comfort level with answering these is different. A standard, "I don't know; I'm so sorry" is always okay because, really, how can you ever begin to answer that?

As a Christian, I have prayed with patients and their families before. Keep in mind, this was only after I had the green light following multiple unprovoked conversations about their beliefs and God's role in their life. So if you feel comfortable and they have given you the green light without you mentioning anything at all first, go for it. I'll never forget those patients; they were so thankful for that support and will always have a place in my heart. Some of my sweetest cards came from these patients.

If you do not practice a religion and the family desires religious comfort, call the chaplain to support them spiritually. Chaplains are an amazing resource and can provide support. Even if the family doesn't identify with that particular denomination or person, the chaplain will know whom to contact to get the right spiritual support.

Your job at this time is to support them, not instantly relieve their emotional pain. Sit with them, comfort them, and empathize with them. I used to feel like I had to come up with the ideal thing to say when someone was crying in front of me, but now I realize that it's not what I say that will comfort them, it's my presence and support, which speak much louder than any words.

Being there for those patients and families is tough, and even if you feel like you haven't helped at all, that's okay. You probably have and had no idea. They'll probably never forget you. They may not remember your name, but they will never forget the nurse who was there for them when their loved one died.

So tell them you're sorry, tell them you're there for them, grab them some tissues, let them cry on your shoulder, hug them, don't be afraid of them, and if they want some prayer from you and you're comfortable with that, go for it. They'll be forever thankful for your support.

Even if you don't know what the heck to say to them, just take really good care of their loved one. That will always be enough, because that's all they want.

Chapter 10

The Shift that Broke Me

Have you ever had a shift after which you didn't know how you'd return to work? I had one of those while I was working in critical care. It literally brought me to my knees it hurt so much. It was a life-changing twelve hours.

I walked into the intensive care unit like any other day. I looked at the assignment sheet and saw I only had one patient. That could only mean one of two things: either God had smiled on me that morning and I only had one patient that day and was open for an admission, or this patient was so time-consuming that one nurse had to take care of only him. It was the latter.

I typically get assigned to the patients who are knocking on death's door and about to walk through it, or the patients with family members who need a lot of emotional attention. I'm not sure if that's a blessing or a curse, but it's part of the job.

I walked over to see an intubated fifty-something gentleman. The family had just stepped out to allow the night shift nurse to give me the report. As the night shift nurse started giving me report, I glanced down at him. I immediately got a shock to my system because he looked a little like my husband. It was also startling because he looked so healthy.

Whenever people are intubated and in the intensive care unit, they usually are swollen, pale, sweating, poorly kept, or have sores, wounds, or abrasions on their face. It is necessary to distance yourself from the situation in order to function as an ICU nurse day in and day out, especially during urgent and emergency situations. This patient took quite a bit more effort for me because he looked like what I picture my husband will look like in twenty years but with a breathing tube. It was quite surreal to see.

The night nurse continued through her report as all of those thoughts swirled around my mind. I tried my best to keep them at bay and pay attention to what she was saying. After all, he was going to be my entire responsibility in a matter of minutes.

He had had a stroke in the worst part of the brain to get one, the brainstem. A blood clot traveled to this area and cut off the blood supply, resulting in an ischemia. You cannot live without your brainstem. It's not like losing your ability to see, speak, or process thoughts normally, as many stroke victims experience. The brainstem is responsible for the most basic and essential functions of the body. It tells your heart to beat, it tells your lungs to breathe.

I looked at him and sighed deeply, thinking about what the next twelve hours would entail. "Today is going to be just terrible," I thought.

Apparently, in the morning he had gone outside to water his plants before work, like he did every single morning, and collapsed. His wife had already left for work, not due to be back until later in the evening. When he didn't show up for work, his coworkers got worried. A friend drove over and found him lying in the yard. After the stroke hit, he had lost all control of his extremities. He was instantly paralyzed and lay there for hours, unable to summon help.

When the emergency medical team arrived at the scene, he was immediately intubated and brought to the hospital, where they quickly tried to retrieve the clot to prevent more damage. It had been so long since it occurred that a lot of damage had already been done. There was nothing that could be done to get back the brain cells that had already died. Once brain cells die, they die. There's no getting back what has already been lost.

That all had happened the day before and overnight he became unstable. Whenever someone has a stroke, the area around the injury typically swells to an unpredictable degree. However, this is not something that occurs immediately. It usually takes some time, anywhere from hours to days, before the swelling sets in. With a stroke in his brain stem, we were particularly concerned about the swelling because of the potential for herniation and subsequent brain death.*

The night nurse was fighting tears giving me the report. She felt like there was something she could have done to prevent it, but there wasn't. We were getting into the territory of what is beyond medicine's ability to fix. It's quite upsetting to watch someone deteriorate right in front of your eyes, when it feels like you should be able to stop it. Attempt to manage your emotions as best you can, and realize that while it may feel like you should be able to help, you can't.

The nurse told me about his wife, who loved him so much. Hearing that just made me nauseous. I couldn't help but think, "You're about to lose the person who has been your best friend for the last twenty-nine years right in front of me and you don't know it yet and I can't stop picturing myself in your shoes."

When his wife walked into the room, I could see how exhausted she was. She had been up for the last thirty-six hours enduring the worst emotional pain she had ever had to endure, and it was taking its toll.

Today wasn't going to be any better.

One minute she was finishing up a conference call, the next she was getting a crash course in neurology. Complex medical language and major medical decisions were coming her way faster than she could handle it.

She walked into the room with a look on her face like she had a knife in her stomach. Sick, in pain, dazed, and confused. She wasn't happy to see a new face this early in the morning and I didn't blame her. With bloodshot eyes, she reluctantly introduced herself to me.

I had completed a full neurological assessment before she arrived and it was about as grim as it could get. He had no basic, primal reflexes. He did not have a cough or gag reflex. He didn't even have a corneal reflex (I could touch his cornea with cotton or saline and he wouldn't even attempt to close his eyes). His pupils were barely reactive. When I opened his eyes, his eyes bobbed downward.[†] They didn't focus on me or anything in the room. Not only did he

---

* **Nursepedia Definition:** *Brain death* is when you no longer have brain function. It is irreversible, and in most states when someone is declared brain dead, they are legally dead. Herniation is when an increase in pressure pushes the blood vessels, CSF, and/or brain away from their usual place in the skull. Brain herniation can result in brain death but not always.

† **Nursepedia Explanation:** When someone's eyes bob and don't track or focus on anyone, it indicates brain stem involvement in their injury, which is a very ominous sign.

not follow any commands with no sedation on board, he didn't respond to any tactile or even painful stimulation. He just laid there, lifeless. He had nothing.

So there he lay with a breathing tube in—no sedation, no reflexes, and no hope for recovery. His wife sat next to his bedside, staring at him. Occasionally she'd run her hand through his hair, looking at him longingly. His sons came in and sat next to him on the bed. One leaned over and started talking to him.

Oh, my heart. I could only observe so much of that interaction at a time without losing it in front of them.

It was going to be a long day.

The phone rang and it was the neurologist. I told him my assessment. He told me that the patient would probably remain in a "locked-in" condition. He wouldn't regain function; he wouldn't progress to brain death. He would just be. He would be dependent on a ventilator forever, if he survived. He would live in a nursing home the rest of his life and never be able to do anything except be aware of what was going on around him without being able to communicate. He would feel pain; he just wouldn't be able to do anything about it. Some people with locked-in syndrome can blink to communicate and breathe on their own, but not him. Too much damage had been done.

"Well, let's get an MRI to see the extent of the damage so I can talk to the family about prognosis and make some decisions today," the neurologist said. I put the order in and let the family know the plan. I made sure not to share with them the neurologist's initial thoughts about the prognosis. I had to keep that to myself because we didn't want to tell them something like that unless we were 100 percent sure.

"I'll take him downstairs to get an MRI, so we can get a really good and detailed picture for the neurologist to go over with you guys," I said to his wife.

She quietly said, "Okay," as she stroked his hand.

I just looked at her as my heart sank into my stomach. I was fighting back tears and it was only 0812. She looked the way I would look if it were my husband in that bed. Her face told me how deeply she loved him. The waiting room, with over forty of his loved ones in it, told me how much everyone else loved him. I tried to compartmentalize all of the thoughts going through my head, because if I was overly emotional, I wouldn't be able to take care of any of them.

"He is my best friend," she said through a fresh batch of tears. "I shouldn't have gone to work. I should have been there."

I didn't know what to say. I didn't know how to respond. I honestly just didn't want to. I wanted to run away and go take care of the patient who was getting ready to go to the floor later in the day, someone who was going to make it out of here. I wasn't prepared for this emotional day.

I sat next to her, putting my hand on her back, and all I could think to say was, "I'm sorry. I am so, so sorry."

After a few minutes, I got up and left her alone with her husband. I went to quickly chart my assessment, grab the meds that were due, and get the monitor I needed to take him downstairs, and then came back. There she was, still staring at him.

While I got things together, people came in and out, all with that same despairing face, the kind of face where you can tell they're using all that's in them not to cry. Their two sons were the worst for me to see, after his wife. One was older (I think mid-twenties, though I'm not sure) and less emotional. He was trying to be strong for his mom and brother.

I packed the patient up and started wheeling him out of the room and off the unit. The patient's longtime friend stopped me, "Can I come down with him? I don't want him to be alone down there."

"Of course you can," I said. "There's an MRI waiting room I'll have you wait in while he's in the scanner."

"Ok, that'll be fine. I just really don't want him to be alone," he said with a quiver in his voice.

He almost got me. Even when I try to have my strongest Nurse Face on, men crying just penetrates my defenses and gets to me. Miraculously, I held it together.

It was a quiet elevator ride and quiet trip to the MRI suite. Normally, I like to make lighthearted small talk when traveling with patients, but not this time. I showed his friend to the waiting room, brought the patient into the room, and greeted the MRI techs.

To get an MRI of the brain, you have to lay flat in the scanner. When you lay down flat, the pressure slightly increases in your brain because of gravity. Not a problem for most patients, but it's a problem for a guy with an acute stroke in his brain stem that we're worried about swelling.

I laid him flat, and initially he was okay. I had an MRI-compatible monitor on him so I could closely monitor his vitals while he was in the scanner.

As I sat there outside the scanning room looking in at his monitor through the large window, I saw his heart rate begin to drop. All of a sudden, his heart rate was 38, his blood pressure was in the 190s, and he was covered in sweat.

"I need to sit him up! He's starting to herniate!" I yelled to the MRI techs as they ran to let me into the room. I sat him up and yelled for someone to grab atropine.* If his heart rate didn't come back up after I relieved the pressure on his brain, we were going to have a brain-dead man on our hands in a matter of moments. Apparently, his brain couldn't handle the small amount of added pressure of lying flat for more than a few minutes. Not a good sign.

Thankfully, his heart rate came back up and his vitals stabilized.

The MRI tech helped me rush him back up to the unit, grabbing his friend on the way. We were not going to be able to get the scan.

I didn't want to explain it all to his friend before I explained it to his wife. As we were walking, I was putting the words together in my mind to tell her what happened and why the scan I told her would take an hour only took nine minutes. I practiced on the patient's friend: "His brain couldn't handle the pressure of lying flat. We won't be able to get a scan on him."

Through tears he asked, "What does that mean?"

"I don't know," I lied. "I have to talk to the neurologist."

As I started getting closer to the unit, his wife saw me and a puzzled look crossed her face as she quickly started walking toward us.

"Let me get him settled and hooked back up to the monitors, and I'll meet you back here to tell you what's going on," I said as she nervously nodded her head. "Someone page neurology STAT for me," I said to the nursing assistant sitting in the nurses station as I wheeled him back to his room.

Another nurse saw me coming back into the unit way earlier than expected and came to ask what happened as she helped me get him back on our monitors.

"His heart rate dropped, pressure skyrocketed, and he got diaphoretic," I told her.

"Oh God," she said. She'd worked in this unit for almost a decade. She knew what that meant. I didn't need to tell her anything else. She told me something ridiculous that another patient did, which calmed my nerves and

---

* **Nursepedia Definition:** *Atropine* is an advanced cardiac life support (ACLS) medication used to increase the heart rate when it drops very low and the patient has symptomatic bradycardia, which can include dizziness, sweating, fainting, and chest pains.

made me forget for a second that I was buttoning up the gown of an almost brain-dead man who looked just like my husband. Thank the Lord for those coworkers who know exactly what to say and when to say it.

The phone rang. It was the neurologist answering my page. I told him what happened in MRI.

"Given the location of the stroke and his assessment, I expected him to be unstable down there. I guess we can't do a scan. I'll be there in about an hour; I'm finishing with a few other patients."

All I could mutter was, "Okay."

I was tired, frustrated, and confused. The emotional ups and downs of the day were already starting to get to me. I was frustrated that I hadn't been warned by the physician, who had apparently suspected this might happen, and confused as to why the scan was ordered in the first place. At this point in the day, getting upset about this wasn't going to provide any relief; it would just make me more frustrated. I took a few deep breaths and put it behind me.

I walked out to his wife who was anxiously awaiting my return just outside the unit in the hallway.

"What happened?" she asked.

I explained to her that I had laid him flat and he'd become unstable because of the pressure in his brain. His heart rate had dropped really low, he'd gotten sweaty, and I'd had to immediately sit him up to relieve the pressure. Because of that, we couldn't get the scan.

"If we just give him some time, can we try again later?" she asked with the last ounce of hope in her eyes.

I paused for a second. I should have told her we needed to wait for the doctor to know for sure. All the, "should haves" continue to run through my mind to this day. I was tired of pretending I didn't know things, tired of seeing that little bit of hope in her eyes.

"No," I said. "And this is just going continue to get worse."

That was it. That's when it hit her that he was gone.

She immediately clung to me and started sobbing into my scrubs. She held onto me so tight, I lost my breath for a moment. Some family and friends ran up to her as soon as they saw her so upset. She was so distraught she almost passed out. I grabbed a chair and she stumbled to it with the help of a few loved ones. With her safely sitting in a chair and her family comforting her

I made a beeline out of there. I was now in survival mode. "If I start sobbing right now, I cannot continue," I thought. I could hear her sobbing loudly as I raced to the restroom, tears filling my eyes and pouring down my cheeks.

The other nurses knew. They knew what was going on. They knew how hard it was for me because they had all seen it themselves. And they, understandably, were just thankful it wasn't them today.

As I got closer to the bathroom, a coworker gave me a reassuring pat on the back. I was thankful for his gesture, even though it made me more emotional.

I closed the door, sat on the nasty bathroom floor, and sobbed. I couldn't hold myself up anymore. I was done. I turned on the water and cried louder. It took about five minutes for me to cry and compose myself. My makeup was gone; I looked like hell, but at that point that was the last thing on my mind. All I cared about was getting through the rest of the shift. I blew my nose one more time, took a few deep breaths, and walked out of the bathroom.

I was heading back to his room to do another assessment and turn him when I saw the neurologist walk onto the floor. We gave each other the "this really sucks" look. I went to go talk with him privately before he spoke with the family, not explaining my frustration with the whole sending me down for an MRI thing, and he said that their options were to let him be locked-in or let him pass. Normally, I would sit in on this conversation to support; however, I was at my emotional breaking point and couldn't take it anymore. I had a feeling I knew what their decision would be and therefore knew how the rest of the day was going to play out and what I would be required to participate in that the doctor would not. I was in survival mode.

I sat this one out.

He took her and a few close family members into the family conference room to deliver the final blow. It took about twenty minutes. I used that time to bathe him, assess him, and just be away from it for a bit to collect myself.

Sometimes these situations come to you with a decision already made. There is too much bleeding, too much swelling, or too much ischemia to sustain life. The physicians have the conversation, letting the family know that the patient will pass. There is no choice involved.

However, there were two options in this situation, and both were rip-your-heart-out terrible.

When you looked at him, he was breathing (because there was a ventilator breathing for him). His heart was beating. He had a blood pressure. Despite the fact that he was comatose, he still looked very alive. You might look at him and think, "Let's just give him some time to come around and see what happens...let's give him a chance." And sometimes, that's perfectly appropriate. But not with this guy. If his family didn't allow him to pass, he was going to be in a nursing home forever, feeling pain, getting bedsores and pneumonia, completely aware but unable to do anything about it. He would not be able to communicate or control his bladder or bowels. He would have a permanent feeding and breathing tube.

I walked back to his room. When I turned the corner into the room, I felt my heart sink to my stomach: There she was, lying in the bed with him, sobbing on his chest.

It ripped my heart out because if I were her, I would have done exactly the same thing. If someone just told me my husband was gone, I'd be lying next to him, sobbing on his chest , knowing that'd be last time I'd lie next to him.

I gave her some time. I had meds and turn due, but that didn't matter. What mattered was that moment, and I was not going to interrupt it.

I came back after a little while to sit and talk with her. She told me stories about him being her best friend and the best father and provider she could have ever hoped and prayed for. Multiple people came in and out, crying. This man had clearly had a profound and positive effect on so many people.

His family members spoke with the neurologist again and decided to let him pass. It was hard to say how long he would last off the breathing tube, so we decided to transfer him to the hospice unit. Typically, we transport the patient from our unit to the hospice unit and remove the breathing tube once we arrive.

We do this because we don't want someone to "fly"* and stay in the busy and loud intensive care unit for days, dying slowly when we thought it was going to be a quick process. Additionally, we don't want to remove the breathing tube before we transfer and have them pass away en route to the next room.

I always dread those cases because taking them down there and leaving them, knowing they'll die, is just really hard.

We secured a bed, and I gave report. The patient's wife, the respiratory therapist, and I walked in silence as we brought him down to the hospice unit.

---

* **Nursepedia Definition:** When a breathing tube is removed and someone does well off the ventilator, we say that they *fly*, like a little bird with tiny wings that you didn't expect to get into the air.

Once we got there, we wheeled him into the room. When his wife, kids, mom, and siblings were in the room and ready, we took his tube out. He was breathing, kind of. I gave his wife and kids hugs and tried not to sob. I wanted to make a quick exit so they could have time alone without some hospital employee looming over them.

As I looked over to get one last glance of him, I saw him take his last breath.

The color immediately drained from his face. I had never seen it happen so quickly. He no longer looked like that perfectly normal guy with a breathing tube. He looked like what little life was left in him had quickly and peacefully slipped away.

I swiftly exited the room for that intimate moment. I could hear the eruption of loud sobs of his loved ones, starting with the people at the bedside and traveling all the way down to those by the nurse's station, as they realized that their husband, father, brother, son, and friend, who had been alive and healthy twenty-four hours ago, was dead. I let out a few tears as I walked by the thirty people in the hallway. I let the hospice nurse know that he'd passed and that his time of death needed to be announced. While I was perfectly capable of doing this myself, I just couldn't take it. I left as quickly as I possibly could.

When I got back up to my unit, it was about twenty minutes from shift change. There was already another patient on the way to take his spot. Thankfully, they would arrive after shift change, and I wouldn't have to take report. I don't know if I could have at that point. I was trying really hard not to cry those last twenty minutes.

Whenever something like that happens, all the other nurses just know. They know the mood in the unit shifts. They know you're on the verge of tears. They know your heart just got ripped out. It's so good to be part of that team because we've all been there. We've all had those patients. And whenever you've had one or the other nurses know you just finished doing something really, really tough, there's this reassuring look they all give you. It's one of those "You're a good nurse, hang in there, we're in this together" looks.

The nurse who had taken care of him the night before was back. I told her what happened and she wanted to go down to hospice with me to see him and the family. I knew it'd be rough, but I felt that it would be good to go see the family one last time.

We went down there and saw everyone. The wife was at his side with a look of peace. She was very calm. His mother sobbed as she hugged me and called me an angel. His brother said thank you through his tears. My coworker and I were just trying to hold it together. We let a few tears sneak out, just enough to keep us from losing it altogether. She was about to work a twelve-hour shift and I had just finished one, and would have to be back again in less than twelve hours.

We walked back and replayed the last twenty-four hours in the elevator. We reassured each other. We supported each other. That situation bonded us greatly. We'd walked through the depths of a family's worst nightmare together.

I went home that night and sobbed on my husband's chest. I cried the tears that I'd been holding in all day. That day, more than any other, I was thankful that his chest was rising and falling as I laid on him, that he could talk to me, that he could walk, and that he could just be.

For the next few weeks, I dreamt about the patient and his family. I saw his face in my dreams with that breathing tube and his bobbing eyes. I saw his wife sobbing on his chest. I felt her cling to me when she found out he was gone. I saw his last breath. I heard his family sob down the hallway.

Sometimes when someone passes, the nurses will try to go to the funeral. I couldn't handle being there, so a few nurses and I sent some flowers.

A week later, my husband and I went to our weekly Bible study. In the women's small group, I shared the situation and started sobbing all over again. One by one, everyone prayed for me. As they did, I felt a release. I felt a peace that I hadn't felt since. I didn't dream about him anymore after that. I felt like God had had a purpose for me in that situation, with that family and wanted to release me of the pain that came with it.

Looking back, I'm thankful I had the privilege of caring for this patient and his family that day, even though it was one of the hardest things I've ever done. I know there was purpose in me being there and am thankful that I could be. I am humbled to be the one that got to be there for them.

I thought that shift was going to break me, and it did. But it broke me in an "I'm so thankful for all that I have" way. It broke me in a way that made me more compassionate, empathetic, and present both physically and emotionally for my family, friends, and patients. Being broken for your patients allows you to enter into what they're experiencing. It enables you to really be present for them and therefore really care for them in the way they need it most, while making sure you're guarding your own heart.

Not only did I learn about being broken for other people, I learned about self-care during these situations. There were many times during that shift when I had to step back so that I could continue to provide care throughout the day. I used to feel ashamed doing this, like I wasn't a good enough nurse if couldn't be all things to my patients and their families all the time. This situation really showed me that I could give all that I *could*, and that would be enough.

Contrary to what I believed before, there's not a certain amount of emotion or tears you need to give to a patient to provide good nursing care. Nurses are people too; we are not these emotional robots who can handle an infinite amount of pain, trauma, suffering, and sorrow, and then provide the exact emotional support to every single patient who needs it, every time. This is why I had to step back at certain points during the day or why sometimes I can't completely go to that emotional place with all of my patients. It is out of self-care and self-preservation that I cannot go there every single time, and that doesn't make me, or any of you reading this, any less of a nurse. It makes you human. Give what you can to your patient, and that will always be enough.

Chapter 11

If It Makes You Feel Any Better

I used to think that good nurses didn't make mistakes. I just assumed that good nurses never messed up. In my head, I pictured someone going into nursing school as a normal person, and if they did it right, they came out as this flawless individual who did not make mistakes because they were a good nurse. I connected the term "good nurse" with "never makes mistakes." Therefore, if you made mistakes, you were a bad nurse.

My goal was to be a good nurse, and therefore, I could never make a mistake.

This expectation is a crushing weight on your chest as a new nurse. It elicits that kind of chest pain that makes you feel like you need some nitroglycerin, morphine, aspirin, and oxygen STAT.

Dispelling the Myth

I want to dispel this unrealistic expectation and thought process, because it can be incredibly frustrating and all-encompassing. You get so focused on not making a mistake that you end up making more. We need to set realistic expectations for new graduate nurses learning how to care for patients.

While nurses do put a lot of effort into doing our jobs perfectly, this doesn't mean we're without flaws. We are human, just like everyone else, and therefore, we will fall short sometimes. Even doctors, who do a really good job of making it seem like they have never messed up, still do at some point.

I think this fixation on mistakes and pretending they don't happen occurs for a few reasons.

1. We want to show our new coworkers that we're amazing nurses.
2. We want our patients to have confidence in us, which can be tough when we're new!
3. We think that if we mess up and admit it, we'll lose our jobs and licenses and therefore our livelihoods.
4. We think that if we mess up, we're not the perfect nurse we always dreamed we would be one day.

Something I've noticed is that many nurses catastrophize even the smallest misstep. We automatically go to the worst-case scenario.

- "I can't believe I gave that guy 50 mg of Lopressor instead of 25 mg. He's going to have a drop in blood pressure, I'm going to have to give him a bunch of meds and send him to the ICU, and the doctors are going to think I'm incompetent and report me. I'll lose my job, get reported to the Board of Nursing, and never work as a nurse again."

- "My patient with an above-the-knee amputation just fell! I thought I did everything I was supposed to do. I think I did everything? The patient is going to report me. My manager is going to report me. I'm going to have to get progressive discipline and be on probation. I'll be the nurse everyone thinks is an idiot who doesn't get even the most basic thing right."

- "I forgot to clamp both sets of tubing when I spiked the unit of blood to prime it. The blood backed up into the saline bag. I'm going to have to throw it all away and start over. She's going to get charged for two bags of blood and sue the hospital for the cost and I'll be liable."

I did all of those things and had all of those thoughts when they happened.

It's incredible how powerful our thoughts are when we're in a situation where we messed something up. It's no wonder people do everything they can to make it seem like they have never made a mistake or try to pass the buck. I get it. When you've convinced yourself that your reputation, job, license, and therefore livelihood are on the line, you will do whatever you can to prevent that from happening.

It is really important to fight this inner battle for the greater good of not only your personal learning and growth but for the overall culture of safety for the unit. You must own up to your mistakes and learn from them to prevent their reoccurrence. Orientation is a time to learn and grow, not a time to constantly perform perfectly. It's hard to learn when you feel like you're in performance mode all the time.

If you mess up, admit it, address it appropriately, and learn from it.

If you don't know something, admit it, ask for help, and learn.

This is how you grow into a safe and good nurse.

Of course, keep the balance in mind; this is not a license to go and flippantly make mistakes with no consequences. Do not be careless or lazy because you're new and therefore extended a bit more grace than usual. However, if you find that you're continuing to make mistakes, maybe you, your preceptor, and your educator need to sit down and really dive into what's going on. There should be a point at which you're not making the same mistakes and are learning, growing, and making progress.

I'd like to dive into some more specific kinds of mistakes, how to avoid them in the first place, and what to do when they happen.

Kinds of Mistakes and How To Avoid Them

There are many different ways you can potentially mess up, some of which are not very obvious. I think it's helpful to be aware of these things first because it can help you avoid them. Most new nurses are familiar with medication mistakes, but mistakes go far beyond that.

Mistake: Drops in communication and assumptions

The health care team is huge and patients are complex, and the nurse is at the center of everything. There are a lot of people to speak to while planning and providing care. Maybe the provider didn't tell you the patient needed to be NPO (nothing to eat or drink) for four hours and took two hours to enter the order. Maybe you forgot you needed to hold the regularly scheduled dose of subcutaneous heparin for surgery later today. Maybe you thought the nurse practitioner was entering the discharge orders, but they actually left for the day. Or maybe the patient told the CNA they needed pain medication but the CNA forgot to tell you, and now the patient is in unmanageable, severe pain and extremely upset at you. There are a lot of things that can be lost in translation.

The most important aspect of nursing is always the patient. In light of this, it is important not to assume that patients understand medical terminology or jargon. Also, the patient may not be familiar with how patient care flows in a hospital. They may not know that in the ICU, their nurse typically cares for two patients at a time, while on the regular nursing floor their nurse could have as many as eight patients, so their expectations need to adjust a bit. They may assume that when the doctor rounds and says, "I'm sending you home!" that means within the hour, rather than in four hours because it takes the nurse three hours to obtain discharge orders from the doctor.

How to avoid drops in communication and assumptions

Round with the physician or advanced practice provider every time they are on your unit. Always touch base with them, even if you don't have something specific to tell them. Ask them if they have any needs or questions for you. Whenever any member of the health care team comes to see your patient, try to be in the room with them if possible. If this can't happen, make sure you touch base with them at some point, either before or after they see your patient. After any health care team member sees your patient, follow up with the patient and ask them how it was in an open-ended way: "So what did the physical therapist have to say today?" After they fill you in, ask if they have any questions or if it all made sense to them. Whenever they verbalize back to you what they understand, make any necessary corrections, and then offer support and encouragement as needed. Create a safe space with your patient in which there are no stupid questions. You want them to feel comfortable enough to let you know when something that seems simple to you doesn't make sense to them.

Along the same lines, it's important not to assume the patient knows all things hospital. I've heard health care providers tell patients that they're NPO, that the patient will be transferred, or that they want to put a line in. This medical jargon is a foreign language to people who don't eat, sleep, and breathe hospital like we do. People may feel silly or stupid asking questions about something that the health care team member presents as obvious, even though they don't really understand.

There are some things that you'll learn with experience. As your critical thinking develops, you'll be able to anticipate needs or things that need to be clarified. Going back to the example of holding heparin before a surgery, in time you'll be able to hear in report that your patient is going to surgery today or tomorrow and instinctively know to peek at the meds due before they leave to ensure they are safe to give preoperatively. You'll know which orders you need further clarification for and be able to anticipate an issue later in the day and manage your time appropriately so that you don't get stuck in an urgent situation that could have been avoided.

Mistake: Failing to plan

It's quite the tall order for the new nurse to hear that a patient needs to go to the operating room (OR), or to dialysis, or needs to have a cardiac cath completed and immediately remember everything they need to do in the order they need to do it. You might think that the nurse would receive a comprehensive to-do list in order to be prepared. Yes, facilities do create preoperative and preprocedure checklists, but they are not all-encompassing. You must frequently facilitate things for which there is no checklist. (Have you clarified all pre-op meds? Were they supposed to have prep last night and did the last nurse make sure to do it? Do you call transport or does pre-op call transport? Who pulls the patient over in the computer, and how do you do it so you don't lose all of your orders?) It truly requires learning each facility's culture and flow to know each little task the nurse must complete.

There is also the time management aspect of this process. Maybe the patient doesn't have a procedure scheduled, but therapy needs to work with them, or they need an MRI and a timed blood draw, or they need consistent pain medication administration or else they'll be in debilitating pain. To get all of these things done, you have to actively plan ahead.

How to avoid failing to plan

When you hear in report that a patient is going to a procedure, you must make sure to touch base with your preceptor to ensure you do all that you can earlier in the shift to have a smooth transition. Do not wait until the patient is leaving the floor to see what needs to be done, or for someone to complain after the fact to understand what should have been done.

You could ask your preceptor (or coworker if you're off orientation), "I see my patient has a CTA ordered later today. Is there anything I need to do to prepare them for that exam?" Additionally, during report, it's helpful to think about what will need to happen during the entire shift for that patient and consider it all at one time. So if you have a timed PTT (prothrombin time) blood draw at 1100 and an MRI scheduled, make sure you're considering that when you're chatting with the folks down in MRI so you don't miss either important task.

Mistake: Medication errors

Medication errors is probably one of the most common categories of potential harm from a nurse. I used to think only bad, clueless nurses made medication mistakes until I made one. While you're trying to give medications throughout the day, there is a lot going on around you. There are multiple points where an error can occur, and the sheer number of meds you are giving is large.

The order could be entered incorrectly, you could forget to cut the pill in half, you could accidentally give two instead of one, someone could interrupt you during your med pass, you could read the sliding scale incorrectly and administer too much insulin, your IV pump could be programmed incorrectly, or the physician might give you a verbal order to discontinue a medication while you're in the middle of giving a bed bath to a morbidly obese vented patient and you forget completely by the time you finish. The point is, med errors happen to even the best of nurses. What is important is how you handle it, what you learn, and how you share it with others so they don't make the same mistake.

How to prevent medication errors

Focus when you're removing medications from the dispenser. Hanging out in the med room is nice. It's one of the few quiet places in the entire hospital, but don't use it to talk to people while you or they are removing medications. Just enjoy the silence.

When you are passing medications, do not allow yourself to be distracted. It can happen very easily: you are passing meds and the physician you've been paging for two hours finally calls back, a family member is on the phone, lab calls with a critical value, another patient has to pee *right now*, the patient you're passing med to will not stop talking, or you've got to get another set of vitals on a patient while they're receiving a unit of blood. It is okay to say, "Hold on, let me finish passing meds, and I will be there." Do not stop in the middle of a med pass to do something that is not an emergency. The physician can hold for another ninety seconds. The family member can call back. You can tell the talkative patient, "Hold on one second, sir. I just need to focus here really quickly while I'm getting your medications situated, and then I'm all ears." I've noticed a lot of patients feel uncomfortable with silence, even if you're clearly concentrating. It is okay to gently remind people that you are focusing, even if it's on a task you could do with your eyes closed.

Make sure you focus while you're programming IV pumps and other equipment, like leveling arterial lines and intracranial pressure monitoring. Many patients don't realize you're either working with a medication (like on an IV pump) or that you messing with those lines directly impacts readings, which affect medications. I honestly feel like I need to focus the most when I'm programming an IV pump, so I find myself asking for a second to concentrate from patients and family members during that time.

I realize nursing isn't a business, but if there's one time for it to be all business with whomever you're interacting with (patient, family, physician, nursing assistant), it's when you're passing meds. Your concentration and focus is the priority to ensure safe administration. You're not being rude or short with someone, you're just all business when trying to focus on meds.

Mistake: Failure to prevent patient injury

You think, "None of my patients will ever fall—ever," or you're sure you'll never have a patient suffer harm under your care, but it happens to some of the best nurses.

While you may have all of your fall-risk interventions in place, maybe the family member turned off the bed alarm and didn't turn it back on before they left. Maybe you forgot to put the call light back on the table, or maybe the sitter fell asleep while watching the patient at risk for suicide (that should never happen, but it can). Patients have a wide variety of things going on with them (such as confusion, meds, pain, a new environment, illnesses, and so forth) at any time, which puts them at an increased risk for injury. While you'd like to have a set of eyes on them constantly, it's not humanly possible unless you've got a sitter for all of your patients around the clock.

How to avoid patient injury

While your physical safeguards against injury are important (call bells, side rails, nonskid socks, and so forth), they cannot be your only means of preventing injury. People will forget to put the nonskid socks back on before ambulating, or the patient will figure out how to turn the bed alarm off (both have happened to me). Because of this, it is important to continually educate the patient and their support system about the importance of compliance. It's not that we don't trust anyone in particular; it's that we don't trust anyone at all. We don't trust ourselves or each other to remember every single thing every time, nor do we trust the patient's disease processes, the effects of pain medication, or the effects of exhaustion. People are not themselves when they're hospitalized. The way to go about educating the patient and their loved ones is with a team mentality. When you're telling the patient and their loved ones about these devices that prevent falls or various injuries, say something like this:

> So while you're in the hospital, even if you feel great, you're at a risk to fall or injure yourself. I've had some patients who felt totally normal hit the deck unexpectedly, so you can't be too careful. I know you're here for _____, but we don't want you to have to stay any longer because you got injured while recovering. We've got a few things in place to help prevent this from happening. While you're out of bed, we want you to wear these nonskid socks. Whenever you need to use the restroom, hit your call bell so we can help you. There's a lot to disconnect and keep in line when you're walking. And I'll also have this bed alarm on so if you do get confused and get out of bed without someone, it lets me know I need to come right away. If you or your loved ones see we forgot any of that, let us know. You won't be picking on us and we won't take it personally. Recovery takes a village, and we want to work together to make that happens as smoothly as possible.

Essentially, it's important to communicate:

1. Why they're at risk
2. What you're doing to prevent it (nonskid socks, bed alarm, etc.)
3. That everyone (the patient, their loved ones, and the health care team) is responsible for this
4. That it's not only okay for them to point out if you missed a step, you encourage them to do so

It's not about someone being right and someone being wrong, it is about everyone holding each other accountable, including the patient and their loved ones. If you start off your shift with this open attitude and communicate about helping each other out, that adds arguably the most important safeguard in injury prevention.

I also want to mention that consistency is key. With so many different interventions to prevent falls and injuries, it is easy to forget one or two. Therefore, I encourage you to have a routine or a little mental checklist before you walk out the door each time to make sure those things are not forgotten in the rush.

Additionally, no matter how alert or "with it" my patients may be, I always make them show me on admission that they know how to use the call bell. For example, when I have a new admission, I'll let them know about the unit in the general welcome and informational spiel. Before I walk out of the room, I say, "Before I leave I just want to make sure that you know what button to hit if you need me. Why don't you go ahead and hit it and we'll make sure that it works?" The patient hits the call bell and together we make sure it works (a few times it hasn't worked, so I immediately knew that I needed to grab a new call bell or reconnect it). I've had a few instances where the patient seemed very with it, but when I had them do this quick demonstration, they could not, and I never would've known that had I not asked them to do it. A patient's inability to use the call bell can result in falls and injuries, because if someone has to go to the bathroom quickly or needs anything else, they have no way of contacting you.

Mistake: Breaching policy

Breaching policy sounds scary and official. It can be very serious or very minor, and honestly there are many breaks in policy that go unnoticed. However, policy should be what guides your practice wherever you work. During your orientation process, as you're learning how to do new things at your facility, your preceptor should be referring to the latest policies and procedures. These are routinely reviewed and edited, so if someone went through orientation twelve years ago and hasn't looked at a policy since, chances are they are not doing something according to the latest policy.

Because the medical and nursing world evolves rapidly, it's essential to be informed about the latest changes to practice. If you have a nurse on your unit who hates change and refuses to adapt their practice based on evidence, steer clear, my new-nurse friend. They are dangerous. If their rationale for how they provide care is "That's how I've always done it," or "That's how I was taught during my orientation," it is not a good rationale. Their orientation could have been over a decade ago, and they could have been taught incorrectly.

The specific policies to notice differ depending on your unit and patient population. During my orientation, the policies on assessment and reassessment, restraints, central venous catheter nursing care, medication administration, and internal urinary catheters were all of particular importance. Those policies were stressed because they could easily be unintentionally breached (not reassessing when you should have, not scrubbing the hub before medication administration, incorrect procedure for replacing a central venous catheter dressing), and being misinformed about them could result in harm to the patient.

How to avoid breaching policy

Here are some personal rules I've come up with through my extensive policy and procedure experience:

1. Always look up policies and procedures as you're learning new things in orientation. Use these to guide whatever you're doing, not what someone is "pretty sure about."

2. Trust no one. Some of the most well-meaning nurses have been misinformed, as have some who sounded very confident and sure of themselves. Always look it up for yourself.

3. Don't let anyone talk you out of looking something up and going by it. If you're pretty sure something isn't right, hit the pause button and go grab the policy.

4. Be on a policy review committee to offer bedside perspective and routinely review policy changes.

What to Do When You Make a Mistake

Remember, it is essential to deal with mistakes head-on. Take a deep breath and get into go mode. Stabilize the patient or provide whatever immediate care is needed.

Then, take another deep breath. Think about the support you need. Do you need to talk to your BFF nurse, the charge nurse, your preceptor, or your mentor? Think about whom you feel comfortable going to and saying, "Hey, I messed up. I don't know what to do next."

You don't need to announce in the middle of the nurses' station that you screwed up. Pull someone you trust aside and tell them exactly what happened. This is an instance where it's really helpful to have a good relationship with your preceptor and a handful of other nurses on the unit. Remember, being a good nurse isn't about being perfect; it's about being able to adapt, learn, and grow in order to provide customized and empathetic patient care. Learning how to do that is messy. Mistakes happen. Keep your head up while you're working to remedy the situation in the moment.

Pull whatever policies are necessary so you know exactly what you need to do. In many instances, you probably need to let the physician or advanced practice provider know. Ensure your documentation reflects what it needs to. You may want to have the person who is helping you get situated double-check your charting.

After the dust has settled, reflect. Don't beat yourself up; simply reflect.

Next, I want to empower you to take ownership. Regardless of how you think your colleagues or patients will view you, own your mistake. While I doubt you were acting maliciously, identify where you could have done better. Something like, "Ok, so I know I should have made sure the medication was infusing before I walked out of the room, but I didn't double check it" is a good example.

Debrief with someone you trust, like a mentor. They may have some comforting and encouraging words. They may also be able to provide some practical advice on how to avoid making the same mistake again.

For example, when I titrated my heparin drip based off of the wrong PTT lab result, I pulled the charge nurse aside and asked her what to do. We grabbed the policy, called the doctor (who was a cardiovascular surgeon—yikes!), ordered a new PTT, and followed the policy. After everything was situated, I went to the nurses' station and had an "I can't believe I just did that" moment with the other nurses. I felt idiotic and alone, surrounded by amazing nurses who, I was sure, had never made a mistake like that. And then something really wonderful happened as I sat there sulking around a bunch of nurses I admired.

Everyone else started talking about things they had messed up and what they'd learned from those mistakes. Some stories were serious and some were funny. Regardless, they were incredibly encouraging.

Being a part of the solution

When you're reflecting on an error, it's important to identify why it happened. While it's important to take responsibility for mistakes and errors, it's also important to ensure that you and your colleagues are set up for success. If there is a system issue that needs to be addressed to prevent others from making the same error, make sure that happens.

How does policy change happen at your hospital? Is there a specific committee who meets to discuss the latest research? Are there any bedside nurses on that committee? If so, this is called shared governance.*

When I participated in shared governance at my previous facility, a nurse shared a story about a patient who needed to be paralyzed with a specific medication emergently. When this nurse went to remove the medication as an

---

* **Nursepedia Definition:** *Shared governance* is a model of nursing practice designed to integrate core values and beliefs that professional practice embraces as a means of achieving quality care. Shared governance models were introduced to improve nurses' work environment, satisfaction, and retention (Anthony 2004).

emergent override from the medication-dispensing machine (because it was not in the code cart), he realized that it was not stocked in the machine. This was really odd, as it was a specialized intensive care unit and normally, most urgent or emergent medications are routinely stocked in these machines.

This significantly delayed patient care, as a nurse had to run to another intensive care unit to pull the medication and run back. The nurse who shared the story took it upon himself to bring this issue to a shared governance meeting in which a pharmacy representative was present, and got the specific med stocked in all intensive care unit medication machines in a matter of weeks.

That is learning from a bad situation and being part of the solution. That is how change occurs. Administration is not at the bedside to see these problems to know they need to be solved; it requires an engaged bedside staff to bring issues to light so they can be addressed. The worst response for someone who goes through an experience like that is to be upset about it but let it go without trying to correct or address it to benefit people in the future. Complaining about the powers that be and not diving into the issue and being a part of the solution is just spinning your wheels. Your expertise and opinion is desperately needed in these situations.

If it makes you feel any better...

When I made that mistake with the PTT and everyone started sharing their own mistakes, it really stopped my worst-case-scenario, beating-myself-up mentality. I thought it might be helpful to share many experiences myself or others had, as well as a few that were submitted by other experienced nurses online. To maintain anonymity, I have written these all in the first person.

- I had mini panic attacks before work.
- I freaked out every time I had to call a doctor.
- I cried in the bathroom the first time a doctor yelled at me.
- I cried in the car on the way home after a terrible day.
- I called a patient's wife his mother.
- I took report on the wrong patient. More than once.
- I had to admit a med error to an attending physician and four of her residents.
- I came in on a day I wasn't scheduled to work because I read the schedule incorrectly.
- I accidentally discharged a patient too early and had to call and instruct them to go to a clinic to get a follow-up BMP (basic metabolic panel) drawn after potassium replacement because I misunderstood the physician's order.

- I stood at the door and watched a patient and his mother scream at each other because I was too scared to do anything about it, while another patient and his family member sat there terrified.
- I had a patient call 911 on me.
- I didn't give the meds a patient needed before getting IV contrast for a CT scan, sending them into acute kidney failure.
- I had to implement an order for "scrotal elevation" on a man with a "scrotum the size of a soccer ball."
- I got yelled at on the phone when I called a doctor for another doctor, while he just stood there, knowing I was being yelled at, and did nothing.
- I've had to digitally disimpact way more patients than I'd like to admit.
- I asked a patient with bilateral above-the-knee amputations where her socks were.
- I didn't tell a nursing assistant that a patient was now NPO for a procedure. The patient ate and couldn't have the procedure done. It was a Friday. Because it wasn't an emergency, the procedure could not be done until Monday. The patient stayed in the hospital all weekend because they ate that one meal.
- I spent an hour doing a complex dressing change just to have the physician come by, rip it off, leave, and not tell me anything.
- I had a patient's elderly husband continually call me "Nurse Good Body" and wink at me all shift.
- I had to dig feces out from under a confused patient's nails because I didn't get to the room in time after they had a bowel movement.
- I stayed late because I hadn't charted a word until 1930 and didn't leave until 2100.
- I gave a patient the wrong narcotic.
- I had nursing assistants be really rude and demeaning to me in front of other coworkers when I was just trying to learn the ropes.
- I gave a pain medication too early.
- I was terrified when I floated for the first time.
- I accidentally piggybacked an antibiotic onto a vasoactive drip because I didn't fully trace the tubing back to where it should be.
- I froze during my first code.
- I delegated to a CNA to discontinue the Foley catheter of a patient in a specific room but didn't say the name of the patient (only the room number). The CNA discontinued the wrong Foley catheter, which had been placed in the OR. The patient had to have another surgery to get it put back in.
- I froze when a patient started coding, though I had been a nurse for years; I had been on vacation and just could not think of the first thing to do.
- I had to tell a doctor that I was calling a code on his patient because he refused to listen to my concerns.
- I survived a shift off of saltines, peanut butter, and ginger ale because I didn't have time to stop.

- I've had two accidental needlesticks.
- I had a patient who was crashing with drips maxed out, and I accidentally paused the drips, causing their pressure to tank.
- I had a patient actively dying with only me in the room because the family couldn't take it. A staff member came in the room to complain about something stupid, and I didn't have the courage to tell her, "Shut up, this woman is dying. Have some respect."
- I wasted a lot of time doing patient care and got behind on my charting because I was too scared to delegate to the tech playing on her phone.
- Very early in my career I told a family member there was hope for recovery right after the doctor just told them there wasn't. (I did not look at the physician's note before talking to them and just connected the little I knew about that specific disease process with that patient.)
- I had to get really assertive with a patient who called me stupid and kept putting her finger in my face. She stopped.
- I trusted my patient who was technically a high fall risk and let her convince me that she could get to the bathroom by herself. She fell.
- I sprayed tube-feeding residual all over my patient and myself because I forgot to flip the stopcock. I've done that at least seventeen times.
- I accidentally pulled out a patient's external pacing wire before it was indicated when he was standing up from the recliner.
- I received an order to insert a feeding tube on a patient and was getting up to get the supplies when the nursing assistant reminded me the patient had major nasal surgery and couldn't have one placed.
- I'm still not the best IV starter in the unit despite years of experience.
- I still ask questions every single day.

Sometimes, I make mistakes. But it's how you deal with them that counts.

Do not be your own worst enemy; be your own (humble) cheerleader. Own your mistakes and empower yourself and others to avoid making them again. Be the change that needs to occur in processes that are not safe or could be optimized. If feelings of insecurity or inadequacy start to creep back in after you have learned and grown from a mistake, actively fight those thoughts. Take those negative thoughts captive—they do not get to steal your joy and peace in your career.

I believe in learning from the mistakes of others. Many nurses have shared with me mistakes they've made over the years, and when they do, I listen intently. I want to learn from their experiences. The following story was submitted so that you may learn from the writer's experience. This was an experience very early in her career. Today, she has been working in critical care for many years, saved many lives, and received multiple national certifications.

My Biggest Mistake

by Melissa Stafford, BSN RN CCRN SCRN

Picture this: New grad nurse with less than one year of experience, doing "charge" on the 1500–2300 shift. One of the nurses on the floor was an licensed practical nurse (LPN, we didn't have many of those).

The patient, a man, had had an esophagogastrectomy due to cancer and was far enough out from surgery to be on our med-surg floor. However, he still had an nasogastric tube, chest tube, epidural, and a Foley. Needless to say, this was a pretty labor-intensive patient for a med-surg unit.

Late that shift, I was asked to give morphine by the LPN, who could not administer narcotics via epidural catheter. I checked the order, dose, time, and everything necessary by policy. Then I gave the medication to the patient as ordered.

Some time later, as I was chatting away at the nurses' station, I saw the LPN listening in from afar. There was something about the way she kept looking at me, so I finally asked if she needed any help. She said, "I think so. That patient you gave the morphine to, his oxygen saturations are about 77 percent."

You can imagine my response! I freaked out, thinking in my head, "Why in the heck did you let me talk so long at the nurses' station and not inter-rupt?" I started running down the hall to the patient's room. Literally running.

I got to the room, and sure enough, he was dusky as can be, with a respi-ratory rate of about six. He wouldn't wake up. I screamed at the LPN to page respiratory for a non-rebreather mask. Meanwhile, I ran back to the Pyxis to get Narcan, with a million questions running through my mind. "Did I give too much morphine? Was it too early to give it?" The questions I was asking myself went on and on.

Keep in mind that this was before the days of rapid response teams and I was the charge nurse. There was literally no one else for me to call, espe-cially that late at night.

I got the Narcan and gave it to the patient. Looking back, I'm pretty sure I didn't give the Narcan properly. I remember giving the entire vial at once rather than administering it in increments after dilution. Needless to say, the patient woke right up and was screaming in pain.

He kept yelling that his stomach hurt. I noticed his NG tube had come out about 3 or 4 inches, so I instinctively pushed it back down. I apologized for his pain and explained that I had to reverse the medicine because he was

(continued)

barely breathing. At this point, his sats were now in the acceptable range, so I left the room to call the CV [cardiovascular] surgery group.

As I recounted the tale to the on-call PA, I got to the point in the story where the patient was complaining of severe abdominal pain and I pushed the NG tube back down. As the words came out of my mouth, my own stomach dropped to my feet. Oh. My. Gosh. I should *not* have done that.

They ordered a STAT chest x-ray and requested I call the intensive care doctors to evaluate the patient while they were en route to the hospital. When I found out which intensivist was on for the night, my stomach dropped yet again. Although this particular physician was good with patients, he was really not nice to nurses, especially us "floor" nurses. He would pretty much treat us all like morons.

Once the chest X-ray was completed and radiology sent up the film (the literal film because this was before everything went digital), he walked into the room and saw that the patient didn't look great. I proceeded to tell him what had happened. To say he was less than thrilled is an understatement. He snatched the film from my hand and held it up to the room lights. I was still very new, but even I could see that the X-ray was awful. You basically couldn't see the patient's lungs because they were all whited out.

The patient was whisked off to the ICU, and I sat down with my head hung low to complete an incident report. I just knew that my pushing the NG tube down caused this whole issue. I knew I was going to get fired: I'd caused a patient harm. I felt very defeated. I drove home from work that night in tears, ready to quit nursing.

The next day, I called a friend of mine who happened to be a cardiovascular nurse practitioner and told her what happened. The tears were flowing.

She told me that advancing the NG tube did not cause the main issue, despite how much I had convinced myself that it had. This patient developed acute respiratory distress syndrome (ARDS), and the morphine had zapped the little respiratory reserve the patient had left. She then proceeded to take the time to calm me down and explain that nurses make mistakes. She told me that I had done the right thing to notify all the necessary people of exactly everything that had transpired. She also explained why advancing the NG tube was bad and what I should have done differently.

She also warned me about the surgeon, and boy was she right. He never approached me about what happened. Instead, he wouldn't look at me. He gave me the silent treatment and would barely speak to me for a very long time after this event.

Fast forward a couple of weeks. The patient finally healed enough to return to the med-surg floor. However, he still wasn't able to eat or drink. Instead, he now had a jejunostomy tube (j-tube) through which he got his feedings. Know why?

Remember the NG tube that I re-advanced when the patient woke up screaming in pain? Well, when I did that, it's very likely that I caused a tear in the surgical anastomosis. So every time the patient tried to drink, it leaked out into his peritoneal cavity.

I was absolutely crushed all over again. I did not want to care for him. I didn't want to have to look him in the face. But I was told by some wise people that I just had to. I had to look him in the face, accept my mistake, and move on. Fortunately, the patient was a very kind man, and he never treated me poorly. He did eventually get better and go home, but I don't know whether or not he was ever able to eat or drink independently again.

To this day, it's still one of the hardest things I've ever gone through as a nurse. This event almost broke me; it absolutely crushed what little self-confidence I had as a new nurse. Truly, I was one step away from bidding farewell to the profession entirely.

Every time I think about this, I am reminded of how thankful I am for that nurse practitioner. *She* is the reason that I got through it and stuck with nursing. I was very fortunate that I had her and a couple other strong nurses who were incredibly supportive of me. They didn't ridicule me or make me feel like a failure. Instead, they helped me learn from my mistake and use it to make myself a better nurse. I pray that someday, I can do the same for someone else.

To Summarize

Do not expect to be perfect. Do what you can to prevent mistakes from occurring. Be accountable for your mistakes, and follow the appropriate procedure when they occur.

Reflect

Debrief

Be a part of the solution if there is a system-wide problem

Release the mistake

Empower others around you to not make the same mistake

Reference

Anthony, M. 2004. "Shared Governance Models: The Theory, Practice, and Evidence." *Online Journal of Issues in Nursing* 9 (1): Manuscript 4. www.nursingworld.org/ MainMenuCategories/ANAMarketplace/ANAPeriodicals/OJIN/TableofContents/ Volume92004/No1Jan04/SharedGovernanceModels.as.

Chapter 12

The Nurse Life

Many new graduate nurses will find themselves working at facilities in which the schedule is shift work. This means typically working twelve hours at a time, three days per week. While this can vary, this schedule is relatively standard. Working three days per week sounds great, but those three days are pretty grueling. If you add on your commute and staying late to chart or finish things up (because when you're new you're not typically very efficient), you're looking at sixteen-hour days or nights.

Add to these long days the fact that the rest of the world functions in the nine-to-five world. You'll find yourself working weekends and holidays, and many of you will find yourselves working night shifts. Rarely do inpatient facilities schedule people to work the same days every week, and on top of that, you have an unpredictable job where you never know what you'll be dealing with when you walk in the door. Those of us who thrive on predictability and routine are left wanting.

Getting used to this new order of life can take some adjustment. This is especially true after finally getting very used to the nursing school schedule. It's wonderful to not have to worry about homework anymore (so incredibly wonderful, drinking-a-butter-beer-with-Hagrid wonderful), but there are still quite a few challenges to this adjustment. I am someone who enjoys routine and a degree of predictability, so it really took some time to acclimate myself to this lifestyle.

After much trial and error, I discovered some things along the way that helped me not only adjust to living this way, but also maximize my time both at home and at work.

The foundation of all of this is intention. It's important to be intentional and not passive with your time both at work and at home, because your time is precious. Being on for twelve to sixteen hours at a time while caring for patients takes a lot of mental energy. It not only takes time to prepare to go in for a shift, it also takes time to recover. If you're consistently not preparing, recovering, or owning your own time, you'll find that it owns you as you just zombie shuffle to and from work. This happens slowly over time as habits build, and if you can start off expecting some of these challenges that come with a major life transition, you'll find yourself in not just the driver's seat, but the NASCAR driver's seat, knowing exactly where you're going and for how long, so that you can get a lot out of the ride. Otherwise, you'll find yourself half paying attention in the backseat while someone else is driving, and you'll get angry when you realize you're being taken somewhere you don't want to go.

Communication with Loved Ones

As you're trying this new lifestyle, think about all of the people you live with and depend on, and who depends on you in your day-to-day life. It is absolutely essential to communicate with them throughout this new transition, as with any new routine. For example, when I was a brand-new nurse, I was also newly married and working the night shift. There were a lot of things that I did not communicate to my husband because I just assumed he already knew what I needed from him. However, that could not have been farther from the truth. I was in the midst of learning a new sleep pattern and a new job, and I didn't even know what I needed, so it was really hard for him to know how to support me.

It might be helpful to have a conversation with your spouse or whoever is in your life as you start your new job. Let them know that this is a very different schedule that you're learning, as well as a really new and stressful job. You'll probably need extra support and have to ask for grace and understanding during this time. There may be days where you forget something that you never forget, like to walk the dog, do a load of laundry, get the kids' lunches together the night before, or set out dinner before you leave. It takes some time to get used to a new routine and have it fit into your existing life and commitments.

Also, if those that you live with are not in the medical field it is sometimes hard for them to understand exactly how tough being a nurse is. When you get home and say you had a bad day, that means different things to different people. To the guy who works as an accountant, that could mean that clients were rude, people didn't meet deadlines, files have been lost, and so forth. To the engineer, this bad day could be that a client was upset and yelling, someone threatened to sue, or a mistake was noted on an important document, which can result in a large financial loss. But to the nurse, a bad day could include your patient dying or helping people walk through their worst nightmare, all while you manage their care and the care of your other patients. It simply is hard for someone who hasn't put on scrubs and seen it to truly understand.

Even though I have been a nurse for quite a while, it wasn't until I started writing about some of my bad days that my husband (who is great at empathizing) really understood what a bad day meant. Something clicked all of a sudden. I'll never forget the look on his face after he read something in particular that I wrote that helped him understand what I go through. I write content for NRSNG.com, and after a blog post that other nurses and I collaborated on, we received a message that thanked us for our detailed description of what it's like to be in nursing school. This person said it saved their marriage. Their spouse had no idea what they were going through and continued to have the same expectations for their day-to-day life that they'd had before this person started nursing school. The information in the blog post opened their spouse's eyes and enabled them to empathize on a level that they couldn't before. It is important to have an initial "we really need to get ready for a change to the flow of our day-to-day life" conversation.

It's also important to have the same expectations. For example, making dinner for the family after a twelve-hour shift is not fun. This also might not work because if you are on day shift, you may not get home until 8:00 pm, when kids are usually in bed. My husband and I worked out a system where if I was working my twelve-hour shift, he would make dinner that night. I made dinner three nights, and typically one night we were at a friend's or family's house or out. So this split the work evenly and I wasn't expected to make a meal after a ridiculously long day.

We also had an understanding that the days that I made dinner he did the dishes, and on the days that he made dinner I did the dishes. It again splits the work and sets expectations. Therefore, it was not like we would eat dinner and there would be a ton of dishes and we would just wait for the other to start. We knew who was responsible for taking care of them. The dishes got done more quickly than before, and there wasn't an underlying level of frustration when the other person would fail to meet an unspoken expectation.

Finally, as you're communicating with your spouse or whoever is in your life, remember how important it is to be slow to anger and quick to forgive. You will probably miscommunicate. Even some of the best communicators mess up and think they clearly communicated one thing when the other person heard something entirely different. I'd like to think that my husband and I are good communicators, but we still miscommunicate sometimes, even after seven years of marriage. Therefore, if you're not sure someone is hearing what you're trying to communicate, say something like, "Tell me what you hear me saying." This offers a nonjudgmental way to check and see if you're on the same page. This also opens a door for you to address any misunderstandings before they turn into something bigger that could have been avoided.

Practical preparation

Like I said, those twelve-hour shifts are pretty long. I would get very frustrated if, on the days that I had those long shifts, I also had to do my laundry, run to the grocery store, or do other errands. After talking with my husband, we decided that the days I had those tough shifts were solely for that job, and we would do our best to plan around those days so that I wasn't running last-minute errands that could've been taken care of at a different time. We were not perfect by any means, but it really helped my mental well-being and decreased my feelings of being overwhelmed knowing that I was not going to be expected to take care of those things when I also had to work. There were times where I did have to run to the grocery store after work or throw a little laundry in because I forgot, but that was the exception and not the rule.

When I was trying to find ways to decrease my unnecessary tasks the days and night before my shifts, I identified a few things that, if I just incorporated a little bit of planning, would result in significantly lower stress levels.

First, I made sure to do my laundry a few days before my next shift. When I was a brand-new nurse, I was still trying to find scrubs that fit, so I only had maybe three total scrub outfits I actually felt good in. This meant I had to do laundry after that third shift every week to have clothes for the next week. I made sure to have my laundry done before I went to bed the night before my first shift of the new week.

I started setting my clothes out the night before to avoid the frantic, early-morning searching for good, nonwrinkled scrubs. I then got into the habit of setting out all three sets of scrubs for the week.

I also decided that I did not like ordering takeout food or going to the hospital cafeteria for lunch. I never knew if I was going have time to facilitate that. It was just a lot easier and more relaxing to go to the breakroom, grab the lunch I brought, and eat, rather than calling in an order and waiting for someone to deliver it or walking the ridiculously long walk to the cafeteria. I started bringing my lunch basically every shift. I noticed quickly that I hated waking up early enough to make a lunch so I started packing my lunch the night before.

I am not a morning person, so anything that I can do to facilitate more sleep while still getting out the door as fast as possible in the morning, I do. I prep the coffee so it turns on by itself, prepack my lunch, and set out my clothes the night before.

Eating Healthy

Twelve-hour, nonstop shifts can be pretty rough on your body. You have to eat well to insure you continue to be healthy and don't gain or lose a lot of weight. Things can be so busy that you forget to eat or don't have time to eat anything. You can go from the time you leave for work (0530–0600ish) until 1300 and not even have a sip of water if you're not thinking about it. After being immersed in nursing unit culture for a few years, I've noticed a few behaviors I engaged in that set me up for failure in the nutrition department.

1. **Eating the donuts, cake, cupcakes, cookies, chocolates, Edible Arrangements, or other treats someone brought and left in the breakroom.**

A very thankful family or patient brings in donuts for the staff as a treat. Or it's someone's birthday. Or we outperformed on something. For whatever reason, there's a box full of sugary treats in the breakroom. Sugary treats are often how people want to say thank you or reward you as a nurse. This would be nice if it was sporadic, but it starts to happen just about weekly.

Since it's been six hours since you've eaten anything and you only have two minutes to consume something and get your blood sugar out of the fifties, you might as well make it count, right? I've been there. I've done that. I'm not going to say you can't have anything like that or lie to you and tell you I didn't do that last week. However, be aware of what you're consuming. One donut quickly turns to two. If you're going to allow yourself a delicious donut, try to consider that when you make other meal and snack choices throughout the day. If you eat sugary treats every time you work, you'll start to crave it with each shift, crash a few hours later, and it's just not nutritious. Before you know it, it'll be hard to go a shift without one. Limit your intake; discipline your mind (as Snape would say) when you see those donuts magically appear in the break room!

2.   Ordering out at work.

One of your coworkers decides they're going to order out and starts making their rounds to see who wants to order as well. I don't know about you, but when I spend money on delicious food, I like to ensure I have the time to enjoy it while it is warm. And just because you've ordered out doesn't mean you get to go eat as soon as it arrives. Rarely do the stars align to allow such a glorious occurrence. I've seen many delicious meals sitting in the breakroom fridge for four hours because the nurse ran into an urgent issue they couldn't stop for, and that twelve-dollar salad is suddenly no longer worth it.

My advice is to just bring your own food and stick to it. You'll spend less money. You'll eat healthier. You'll hopefully be able to enjoy your entire break. And you won't have to stress about getting to lunch whenever the food arrives. Then when you actually spend the money to eat out, you'll be able to enjoy it, and it'll be more of a treat.

Am I saying I've never eaten out at work or telling you never to do so? No way! I would save the times for ordering out for special occasions, like a birthday or someone's last day. That way you can be part of the team without constantly spending money and eating whatever sounds good at the time instead of what's good for you.

3.   Not preparing.

As I previously stated, unless extenuating circumstances present themselves, I always bring my lunch. I like to plan lunches I really look forward to, so it doesn't feel like I am punishing myself by not eating out every shift.

However, there are those times when a shift was really rough, or something happened at home so you got to bed way too late so making your lunch for the next shift simply isn't happening. To prepare for these circumstances, I allot myself a certain amount to spend on whatever I want at work. If someone is running down to the nice coffee kiosk, people are ordering out for the NP's birthday, last night was crazy, or some other uncommon circumstance occurs—I order out. This keeps me from overspending and also from feeling like I can't ever get anything at work. Balance is key.

4.   Not snacking during the day or consistently at night.

When I talk about packing my lunch, I don't just mean one meal. A twelve-hour shift is a really long time, and one meal isn't going to cut it for me. Also, I find that whenever I wake up before my shift, rarely am I hungry enough to eat breakfast. I am usually really hungry about two hours before the end of my shift. Therefore, I make sure to bring additional snacks to get me through these hungry times of the day.

I like to have something kind of quick, in case I don't have enough time to heat something up or prepare it. A piece of fruit, a protein shake, nuts, a granola bar, and meat and cheese slices are some examples.

On day shift, I enjoy a snack after I finish my morning med pass, eat lunch as close to 1200 or 1300 as possible, and then have another snack around 1600 or 1700.

On night shift, I enjoy a snack after my evening med pass, eat dinner around midnight, and have a snack around 0300.

Also, when I started out, most nurses didn't go to lunch until 1400 or after, even though most had a bit of a lull around 1230 and had time to do so. We almost wore this "I ate lunch late" merit badge. And then one nurse started taking lunch at 1230 and the culture shifted. People started going to lunch when they had time, not when they thought it was socially acceptable to go. We started getting lunches done earlier and people were less grumpy and stressed.

5.   Forgetting to drink water, or only drinking soda, coffee, or energy drinks.

Running around a nursing unit is exhausting. It can truly feel like a twelve-hour workout sometimes. Staying hydrated is essential. I bought a water bottle I really liked and try to drink and refill it three times in one shift. I limited myself to one coffee in the morning and one in the afternoon, although there are many times those cups of coffee sit in the breakroom, getting cold because I simply don't have time to drink them.

Drinking water is essential to health, especially when you're working hard as a nurse. Those energy drinks, coffees, and sodas will only slow you down and make you feel worse overall. Your body desperately needs water, but if you drink these instead, it has to process all the sugar and ingredients that accompany them. I started out allowing myself a soda each shift, because I love soda, I was working hard, and that's only three a week, right? Well, not only did I start to gain weight, I also started to depend on them for energy, and my desire for one each shift simply got stronger. I switched to coffee with one or two sugar packets. This means I went from consuming 124 grams of sugar a week from sodas to 15–30 grams a week in my coffee. The recommended daily allowance of sugar is 25 grams and each of my cherry Pepsis were 42 grams, which is getting close to double my entire daily amount in one drink.

Meal planning

My husband and I are big meal planners, and I love it more than getting a flashback in an angiocath when I'm starting an IV. Once a week, we sit down and look at our schedule for the upcoming week and decide who will make dinner on which nights and what we'll have. We then make our grocery list based on that and our normal breakfast, lunch, and snacking needs. We inevitably miss something, but we are at the grocery store only one or two times per week, instead of four or five times per week, like we were before we started planning meals.

I don't know about you, but I don't mind making dinner. I actually enjoy cooking. However, I loathe figuring out what to make. I like having a plan for our meals, but sitting down to figure them out gives me a tiny myocardial infarction each time. I hate it, but I love that we can have the whole week planned out in a matter of five minutes. That daily headache of looking to see what we have, thinking about what sounds good, and then making it is gone.

Whenever my husband and I are going to bed, we look at what's for dinner the next day and pull whatever is needed out of the freezer and put it in the fridge for the meal. Our meat is defrosted and ready to go by the time we start cooking, and we're thinking about what we're making all day. If it's something I really like, I'm excited, and if it's something that's not my favorite, at least I know it's coming and I don't have that let down at the end of the day: "Ugh. I guess we'll have this stupid casserole today." It's kind of like when you know you've got to take your patient to MRI later in the shift. I am not excited about it overall, but because I know it's coming I can mentally prepare for it rather than all of a sudden getting an MRI order and having no time to mentally plan.

Activity

Making sure you get exercise is really important. I know that is a pretty standard thing I'm sure you were expecting to hear. It was kind of hard for me to adjust my workout schedule to my nurse life schedule. I previously tried to work out five times per week, which meant that some of the days I worked at the hospital I had to come home and work out. Well, that didn't last long. I was simply too mentally and physically exhausted to work out before or after my shift.

I did finally figure out a routine that was a very practical way to go about ensuring I got my workout in. I started working out three days per week instead of four or five. One of those three days would be more cardio focused, while the other two would be more weightlifting focused. All three days consisted of good back and abdominal exercises. This enabled me to work at the hospital three days, work out three days, and have one day off completely. This was the most sustainable routine for me while working at the bedside. It was important for me to get into a habit I could continue for a long time, because following a really intense and exhausting workout schedule for a short period of time may have been helpful then, but what mattered was what I was going to continue to do week after week, month after month, and year after year. Sustainability is key; you are creating a lifestyle, not a short-term fix.

Customize Your Care Plan

I was an athlete in college, so you would think I would enjoy getting in a workout. To be honest, I really do not enjoy working out in the gym much. I spent quite a bit of time pretending that I enjoyed working out because as a former athlete, I thought I was supposed to. But I got tired of pretending and started to ask myself why I felt the need to.

I decided that I had to figure out what worked for me and my schedule—not my husband's, my friend's, or the people I worked with who were in really great shape and talked about these really intense workouts they did before each shift. When you overhear that stuff, it can send your mind to an unhealthy place where you think you have to do what they're doing and do it better, or do something more intense just to be a part of the conversation and not feel bad about yourself.

I want to do something because I know it's good for me and gives me some time to be by myself in this ever-noisy world. But, if I could be just as healthy and never work out, I would most definitely do that. Some people really enjoy working out, doing really intense outdoor activities, or practicing yoga or Pilates. I just encourage you to try different things to figure out what works for you and what makes you feel healthy, not what the most fit and active person on your unit does.

There is no one-size-fits-all kind of approach to exercise and working out. What works for someone willing to get up at 0400 daily to run seventeen miles does not work for me.

Everyone's mind, body, life situation, and commitments are different, and just because I don't enjoy doing what someone else who is super into working out enjoys doesn't mean I'm less than them. I enjoy various things, but running marathons is not one of them. At the end of the day, it is essential to think about what would be best for you, your body, and your schedule and then unapologetically go for it because it is best for you.

While you're figuring out all of this for you and your life, it is essential to acquire a baseline understanding of what healthy eating and working out looks like. Then it's up to you to figure out how you can fit that in with your life.

One of my favorite sources for information on nutrition is the Authority Nutrition Blog (https://authoritynutrition.com). It's an evidence-based approach to the latest research on nutrition (nerding out over here about evidence-based practice!). I haven't found an exercise equivalent, but I think it's essential when you are figuring out what kind of routine you want to get into to check out some of the latest research.

Throughout nursing school, you learn ways to look up research articles and what makes something a reliable study, so I encourage you to use that knowledge to research what you'd like to see if it truly is a good and sustainable option. Sustainability relates to not only your physical ability to get through the workout, but to your ability to continue the routine. What's the likelihood for injury? For example, if your workout is focused solely on running for forty-five minutes three to five times a week, likely to cause an injury, or requires an expensive gym membership, you must consider whether you'll be able to keep up financially.

Another thing that is really helpful regardless of the plan you come up with is having an accountability partner. My husband and I do that for each other. When he notices I'm slacking on working out, or I notice that about him, or we notice the other needs a little extra motivation, we talk about it. It is really helpful to try to eat well and care for yourself along with someone else, instead of out on your own. It's also incredibly hard to eat healthy if the person you share meals and groceries with is not.

Night Shift Tips

Working night shift can be tough on your body, especially when you're doing it for the first time at a brand-new, intense job. In addition to figuring out how to eat properly, I had to figure out how to maximize my time off on night shift so that I was not a zombie when I woke up. It took my body a while to adjust. Here are some hints to getting good, continuous sleep during the day while living the nocturnal life.

1.   Buy good blackout curtains.

These will be a worthwhile investment. You will need to sleep in a quiet, dark environment during the day. I bought some great ones online that weren't too expensive. Keep in mind that short of sleeping in a room with no windows, there's no way to completely block the light. Unless you secure a blackout shade to the wall, light will come through. Please don't go into a hypertensive crisis like I did when I put some up for the first time.

2.   Get a good fan or something with white noise to drown out the sounds of the day.

Someone will start to mow their lawn, someone will come home and acciden-tally slam the front door, or your dogs will bark. You must prepare to drown out sounds because it will not be silent in the middle of the day unless you live alone with no other homes or buildings for miles. I kept a fan on, which really helped. You can also purchase a cheap sound machine that will get the job done. There's no need to pay hundreds of dollars for a fancy one; there are definitely cost-effective options.

3.   Turn off your ringer on your cellphone and just have an alarm on.

People will forget what days you work and that you sleep during the day. The last thing you want is to have your precious sleep interrupted because some friend wanted to text you yet another meme at noon. I actually got a home phone line and only share that number with work and my close friends and family. Work only calls to let me know to come in if I'm on call, and my friends and family could reach me on that phone in an emergency. I am notorious for losing my cell phone, and the peace of mind I have from always having a landline is well worth the $10 per month.

4.   Have a routine with your spouse or roommate(s).

My husband intermittently works nights as well, and we talked about what would best help the other person who is trying to sleep during the day. Even really little considerations go a long way. Things like keeping the shades drawn during the day so the dogs don't bark, setting out clothes, showering in the guest bathroom after a workout, and touching base about what time we want dinner before going to bed that day all made a huge difference. When I worked nights for a long period of time, I actually kept some clothes in the guest room so I could shower and unwind after a shift before he woke up and vice versa. These small changes allowed both of us to maximize our sleep, making us less grumpy when we were around each other.

5.   **Talk to your doctor if needed.**

This is important if you're starting nights for the first time and you take multiple medications. You may need to come up with a new plan for when you'll take your meds to optimize their effectiveness. Your physician may also have some input on other helpful changes to make, specific to your needs.

6.   **Have some snacks that you can quickly eat when you wake up starving at 1200.**

It never failed. I would always wake up around 1200 ravenous every single day that I slept. I just wanted to quickly eat something and head back to bed. If I didn't have anything healthy to eat, I'd eat junk. I looked like Johnny Depp in *Secret Window*, cramming Doritos into my face as fast as humanly possible. Whether this is a premade protein shake, some fresh fruit or veggies, some raw nuts, or a granola bar, it's very helpful to be ready for this before it happens.

How to "flip" for night shift

The hardest part for me about working nights was figuring out how to coordinate my sleep schedule so that I was functional on my days off. I've talked to quite a few night shift nurses, and there seem to be three main ways to do this. Some people "flip" every single day (go back to being awake during the day, asleep at night), some only flip if they have more than one day off, and some never flip (always awake at night and asleep during the day). It all depends on what you want to do and what fits with the rest of your life commitments.

I'm going to go through my general process for flipping. If you never flip, this doesn't apply. You're just awake at night and asleep during the day. If you flip every day you have off, you stay up after you clock out and wait to go to bed until that night. I could never handle that because I would fall asleep around 1100, sleep until 2000, and be wide awake all night.

Let's say I'm working Monday, Tuesday, and Friday. To prepare to be up all night, I stay up until at least 0200 on Sunday. I then go to sleep until about 0900. When I got up, I'd get some light stuff done around the house or do something low-energy that I enjoyed, and then take about a two-hour afternoon nap. After this, I would get up, get ready, and go to work.

I'm not a heavy coffee drinker—if I have more than two cups, I'm tachycardic and hypertensive. So I space them out, drinking one cup on my way to work and one cup at 0200. If it's past 0300, I stay away from the coffee so I can go to sleep when I get home.

Monday to Tuesday is easy because I go to bed as soon as I get home and wake up around 1700 to eat my dinner and head to work.

When I get off work Wednesday morning, I go to bed immediately when I get home. I set an alarm for 1200 or 1300. I may be exhausted, but I force myself to get up and drink some coffee. Then, I go to bed at a normal time that night and consider myself "flipped." I sleep that entire night, usually getting up pretty early the next morning, ready to enjoy my day off. I then prepare for my Friday shift like I did for my Sunday shift.

If I only have one day off in between workdays, I don't flip. It's just too much effort for my sleepy head to go through. I know some people who do and it works for them, but it's too much for me.

There is also another option: sleeping from about 0200 to 1000 on your days off, which enables you to have a foot in the day world and a foot in the night world. You're able to participate in some things during the day without totally altering your sleep schedule.

Rules of engagement

I know what you're thinking—this is a lot of rules to live by. However, I did not figure this stuff out overnight. I'm telling you how I've fine-tuned my routine through quite a bit of trial and error. I had to mess up a bunch to figure out that this is what works for me.

It does sound like a lot to think about every single day, but I've found that if I have a routine, I just feel better overall and have better control over my life. I don't just order food based on what I'm craving, or grab a soda because I want to. I eat what I bring and don't give myself the option to eat something else. I make sure to have all of my stuff together and organized so I won't have to take a thirty-minute trip to the grocery store after a horrendous fourteen-hour shift. I don't compromise my sleep schedule for anything unless it's very urgent or an emergency. Along with the support of my husband and the understanding of loved ones, this is not only possible, but also very doable and sustainable.

Working these long twelve-hour shifts can get a little depressing, especially if it means you miss out on some stuff in the rest of your life. The more active role I have in my little every-day decisions make such a difference. It's important to feel like I am in the driver's seat of my life and not in the back-seat just watching what happens. This doesn't mean that I never unknowingly run into something or have to deal with a flat tire at times, but generally I am in control of my life and decisions.

Starting out with control over your eating, sleeping, and living choices, as well as not giving yourself the option to do poorly, will hopefully make things easier. It's hard to avoid just eating and drinking whatever you want in this shift life. That behavior is hard to break after years of sitting in the backseat.

Does this mean I am crazy strict all the time and hate my life because of the rules? No. It can get a little daunting, but the overall result and control is better than the freedom to eat anything and everything. Eating and doing whatever you want without any plan or thought of the big picture becomes harder to control over time, so it isn't a freedom anymore. I'll have a slice of cake during nurse's week, a cookie or two if someone brings them, and defi-nitely a donut (I *love* good donuts) once in a while. But I don't order pizza one night, Chinese the next, and McDonald's the next, and have cookies, cakes, and soda for regular everyday snacks. That is simply unsustainable.

The first few months of night shift were incredibly challenging for me and my husband. Not only was I new to night shift, but we were also newly married. We were still learning how to live life together. I lost my cool and flipped out on him for being so incredibly loud during the day, though he actually was not being loud at all and was trying to be quiet. I was being dramatic and having trouble controlling my emotions from the stress of work and lack of sleep, and I had not communicated my expectations for how I needed him to support me while going through this transition. Doing so removed a huge burden of stress and festering frustration from us both, and in turn, we were happier and more satisfied with our jobs and marriage than before.

Work-life balance is important no matter the profession. When working nights or twelve-hour shifts, you have to take a more active role to maintain a healthy work-life balance, because it's so easy to just stop trying. For some people, this comes naturally. However, that wasn't the case with me. I had to work at it, figure it out over time, hold myself accountable, and let my husband in on everything, approaching life with a team mentality. I cannot begin to explain how important it is to make sure the people or person you live with knows what lifestyle habits you need to have to maintain a healthy work-life balance.

Figuring out your work-life balance

I think the foundation of work-life balance is truly being all-in wherever you are. This means that you're mentally at the top of your game so you can fully enjoy your time off, however that may look, and you are also focused when you are at work.

Being at this point mentally requires knowing yourself and what you need, which isn't always straightforward. Rest is important, but simply getting good sleep doesn't fully mentally prepare you to walk into work and care for people who are going through trauma, walking through their worst nightmare, or bringing new life into the world.

I'd like to walk you through what getting mentally prepared looks like for me.

The spiritual side of my life is incredibly important to me. When nonnurses say, "I have no idea how you do this," my mind always goes to God. That is how I do this.

I pray on my way to work to get my mind right. I pray for peace, strength, discernment, and just to be a good nurse and coworker. Truly, I believe that the reason I can walk into this stressful and emotional job with peace and joy every single day is because God gives that so graciously to me. I thank Jesus for his sacrifice. I thank him that I have a job, that I have my health, that I can breathe, walk on my own, and make my own decisions. Working with stroke patients who suddenly lose basic functions constantly keeps this on the forefront of my mind.

Whenever you're new and in this constant state of learning, doing, and going it can be easy to forget your "why," your "how you do what you do." It may be beneficial to center your mind on your purpose as you commute to work. Everyone's "why" may look different, and sometimes figuring it out can take some soul-searching. Regardless, I highly recommend taking some time to identify what that means for you and bringing your mind back to that place before each shift. It can help put things in perspective, as you walk through some really challenging experiences as a nurse.

It's hard sometimes for that gut-wrenching reality not to take over my thoughts. I don't know if any one reading this ever struggles with being too aware of the fragility of life. It is definitely a struggle I have had, especially after working in intensive care. My mind started to get into "worst-case scenario" thinking all the time. I just assumed all of my loved ones would die an ugly ICU death or a sudden emergency-department death. While prayer was really important in keeping me from going too far with that fear, what really helped shift my mentality was something Dr. Brene Brown, research professor at the University of Houston Graduate College of Social Work and author, said.

The term she uses for this constant dress rehearsal for emotional tragedy is "foreboding joy." She discusses it in-depth in her book *Daring Greatly*, which I highly recommend. When you feel yourself experiencing foreboding, she encourages you to lean into gratitude. I started doing this whenever I find myself mentally going into these worst-case scenarios. When I start to go there, I dive head first into thankfulness. Whenever I picture my daughter coding, I stop myself and focus my heart and soul on just being thankful for her existence and giving her a few extra cuddles. Whenever I picture my husband intubated, I take a deep breath and remind myself of how thankful I am that he's breathing on his own right now. It makes me so thankful for now, because tomorrow is not promised. (Truly, if nursing teaches you something, it's that each day with your loved ones is a gift.) It helps me mentally get back to where I need to be to be present right now.

I'm grateful to Dr. Brown for helping me enjoy every day with my loved ones. If I had not read her book when I did, I am not sure where my mental state as a nurse would be. I had a thankful heart before, but leaning into gratitude during those critical vulnerable moments has been life-changing.

It is essential for me throughout the challenging shifts that come up every so often to try to do the best I can with what I've been given while I'm there. That allows me mentally to "leave it all on the court," as the saying goes. I do the best I can, and if I've done that, there's no use worrying or stressing about what more I could have done. I take care of my patients and their loved ones like they are my family, and really, that's all anyone can ask you to do. So when I am at work, I am truly focused on their needs.

I try to handle mistakes the way I described in the previous chapter. I try to communicate well throughout my shift with everyone from the housekeeper, to the patient, to the physician. I give others grace and try to extend the same to myself. No one is perfect; we miscommunicate, drop the ball, and mess up. Learning how to handle that for myself and how to support others when they mess up has been incredibly powerful.

As you are learning how things flow, getting more efficient and more comfortable in your new role, there will come a day when you cross over from novice to advanced beginner. That point in your career is extremely pivotal. It's so important that I wrote another book about it. To give you a short explanation—essentially this point in your career is when you can either dig deeper into nursing and what you're passionate about, or you can start to become complacent. Once you conquer the challenge of advancing from novice to advanced beginner, I encourage you to take a mental breather. Maybe take a vacation or some personal days to just high-five yourself for getting to that point because it is a challenging journey. Once you recenter yourself, it is essential to continue challenging yourself to prevent complacency. A unit of complacent and grumpy nurses is awful to be a nurse on, but even worse to be a patient in.

Diving deeper into nursing looks different for everyone. Nursing is an incredibly large profession with many amazing options. I wrote *What's Next? The Smart Nurses Guide to Your Dream Career* about this to really spell all of those options out, because it took me time to put all of those pieces together for myself. I spent some time spinning my wheels because I didn't really know what to do next.

Conversely, when I'm at home, I try to be present at home. Turning off my phone to just being there and enjoy the moments with loved ones really makes them more rewarding and memorable. I found myself oftentimes being half-present, mindlessly scrolling on my iPhone when we were supposed to be enjoying a movie together or constantly connecting whatever we were talking about back to work. To avoid this and really be present at home, I found I needed to do two things. First, I need to set aside a little time for me to mindlessly scroll through my phone after a tough day. I just need a silent breather to unclench. After all of those constant beeps, buzzes, and phone calls, I just need some time to enjoy silence and whatever I enjoy looking at on my phone. I typically like checking out what happened on Twitter or Instagram, the news for the day, or what people posted on Tumblr. It's kind of like that sitcom husband who just needs a moment of peace after he gets home from work. I feel like I just need twenty minutes after I change out of my nasty work clothes to sit on my bed and silently scroll.

Second, I really need to debrief my day to someone. Oftentimes I call my mom to talk about my day on the way home from work to exhale out all of my emotions from the day. After twelve hours of keeping a Nurse Face on, it is really therapeutic to let it all out to someone in order to let go of it.

Sometimes I chat with my husband about it as well. By doing this, I'm not still hanging on to underlying frustration from the day hours after the shift.

This is important because if I don't do this, I'll still be thinking about the shift three hours later when I'm trying to enjoy time with my husband or friends, and then I really am not enjoying time with them, I am simply there. Being physically somewhere and being present are two different things, and if I don't processing my day at all, I won't be mentally present. This leaves me feeling like I have an emotional hangover from work, but am not emotionally fulfilled at home. Unresolved feelings of frustration, anger, grief, sadness, or even happiness and excitement are sort of left to stew and not be expressed. I need to process my day with someone to fully allow myself to experience all those emotions, to feel fulfilled both at home and at work. If I don't deal with it and am only half present, not only do I suffer but so do my husband and the people around me.

To enable you to figure out your own work-life balance, I want to encourage you to communicate, plan, eat right, exercise, take time off, and hold yourself accountable for your decisions every day. Be intentional with how you go about your day and your life. Be mentally present at work and at home, figure out what it is you need practically and emotionally for this to happen, and advocate for yourself.

This will enable you to be all in wherever you are and gives you control over your life. You will find it easier to make the right decisions during stressful and compromising situations. Remember, adjusting to the nurse life isn't easy. There will be bumps in the road. Adjusting to this new life role and getting your body used to shift work is challenging. Be quick to communicate and quick to forgive, prepare practically and mentally, take negative and self-defeating thoughts captive, respond to foreboding joy with gratitude, and be ever so slow to anger with those around you.

Figuring all of this out is a journey, especially when new seasons of life begin, like starting a family, moving, or switching jobs and schedules. Give yourself grace as you work through the kinks and grow as not only a nurse, but as a person.

Thank You and Welcome to Nursing

If you're in nursing school, are currently a nurse, or are a retired nurse— thank you. Thank you for what you do or have done. Not everyone has nursing within them. This profession truly requires emotional intelligence and an ability to dive deep within yourself to be all you can for others who are experiencing trauma, crisis, stress, and major life events—and that's just a normal day at work!

This career truly requires all of you and taps into parts of your hearts and lives that most are not okay with sharing. Thank you for going there. Thank you for *being* there, holding someone's hand as they pass away because their family couldn't get there in time. Thank you for spending time with the teenager dying from cancer. Thank you for delivering that baby because the doctor didn't get there fast enough. Thank you for allowing people to die with dignity. Just thank you.

I am honored to be a nurse along with you. It brings me great joy to be able to help you grow as a nurse. I pray this book helped you and that it will help you help others. I pray that you are more confident not only in your nursing skills, but also in yourself. You are a precious commodity, nurse-friend of mine. Please take care of your body, mind, and soul, however that may look for you.

Welcome to nursing. I hope you profoundly impact not only the patients you care for, but also your colleagues with whom you work, and the profession as a whole. Regardless of what you do with your nursing degree, you have the power to impact many in profound ways.

I would like to conclude this book by tipping my nursing hat to you.

Stay humble
Stay confident
Stay strong
Never stop learning!

Recommended Reading

Admit One: What You Must Know When Going to the Hospital, but No One Actually Tells You by Kati Kleber

Being Mortal: Medicine and What Matters in the End by Atul Gawande

Code of Ethics with Interpretive Statements by the American Nurses Association

Critical Care: A New Nurse Faces Life, Death and Everything in Between by Theresa Brown

Daring Greatly: How the Courage to Be Vulnerable Transforms the Way We Live, Love, Parent and Lead by Brene Brown

From Surviving to Thriving: Navigating the First Year of Professional Nursing Practice by Judy Boychuk Duchscher

I Wasn't Strong Like This When I Started: True Stories of Becoming a Nurse by Lee Gutkind

The Nerdy Nurse's Guide to Technology by Brittney Wilson

Nursing School Thrive Guide by Maureen Osuna

The Shift: One Nurse, Twelve Hours, Four Patient's Lives by Theresa Brown

Test Success: Test-Taking Techniques for Beginning Nursing Students by Patricia Nugent

What's Next? The Smart Nurse's Guide to Your Dream Career by Kati Kleber

When Breath becomes Air by Paul Kanalithi

Your Last Nursing Class: How to Land Your First Nursing Job by Beth Hawkes

Talking Points Examples

Sometimes, I know what I really want to say but just don't have the words to communicate it successfully. It's kind of embarrassing if I don't know, especially if it's something simple. It can be tough to effectively communicate when emotions are high, patients are not doing well, and you're trying to do a thousand things at once. That's why I'm a huge fan of talking points. I took all of the ones mentioned throughout the book and listed them here for easy reference. Enjoy!

Introducing yourself to staff during clinicals

"I'm new to this whole clinical thing and want to be as helpful as possible, so if there's anything I can help you with or anything that needs to be done, please tell me. I may not realize some of the things that need to be done yet"

Clarifying communication

"What I heard you say is _____. Is that correct?"

Introducing yourself to members of the health care team

Physical therapist: "Hey, can I see Mr. Smith in 82?"

Me: "Hi, I'm Kati. It's nice to meet you. I'm actually a new nurse and not sure what kind of information you need typically. Can you let me know what you're looking to know specifically about Mr. Smith for an update?"

Physical therapist: "Oh yeah, sure. I'm Josh by the way. I just need to know how he's doing getting out of bed, if it's clinically appropriate for me to see him, and if he's been walking twice a day and up to the chair for meals."

Seeing if a patient would like to speak with a chaplain

"Would you like to chat with someone and process this information? I know it can be pretty overwhelming and sometimes it's helpful to talk about it with someone outside of the situation. Gloria, our chaplain, is a great sounding board and trained counselor. Would you like me to see if she has some time to come by?"

Talking to a patient about pain control

"So, typically when a patient has a pacemaker placed, it's a procedure with minimal pain involved afterward, and the pain that remains is usually controlled with oral pain medications. I want to make sure that your pain is controlled, that you're getting the support you need, and that something else isn't going on with you medically. If you don't take anything recreationally and require this much pain medication, that is a bit of a red flag that there may be a bigger problem from the surgery. I really want to make sure I know what's going on. If you've got a tolerance or dependence, that's a different matter. We can chat together about the best way to handle that, but it's really important I just know what we're dealing with so we can come up with the best plan to maximize pain control and healing."

Polite ways to ensure the off-going nurse hasn't left you hanging

"Oh, and if you could hang a new bag of Levophed before you leave, that'd be great. Thanks."

"Can you give that heparin shot that was due at 0600 before you take off? Thanks."

"Their blood sugar was due an hour ago; if you could grab that before you leave, I'd really appreciate it."

Communicating your priorities to others

"I hear that you need _____ right now, and I will address that as soon as I finish with this priority. Thanks for letting me know."

"I have some very pressing patient needs right now. I will get to that as soon as humanly possible."

"Thank you for letting me know—I will be there as soon as I can, after I'm done taking care of what I'm dealing with right now."

Apologizing to patients for something out of your control

Instead of: "Sorry it's taken so long for me to get here. We're so short-staffed today it's not even funny!"

Try: "I'm really sorry it took a while for me to get your medication. How have you been feeling? Is there anything I can get for you while I'm here?"

Introducing yourself, communicating your time management to your patients

"Hi, my name is Kati and I'll be your nurse today. Today, we have an MRI scheduled, and it looks like I'll be drawing some blood around lunchtime and again around dinner. I'll explain a little bit more about the MRI later. If those labs come back where we need them to be, we could be looking at discharge tomorrow. I'll be back in about thirty to forty minutes to bring some more morning medications and do an assessment. Is there anything you need right now?"

"Alright Mr. Jones, I am going to get report on my other patients now. Is there anything I can grab for you? I'll be back in about an hour to bring some medications and do my assessment."

"I'll be in to give your medications and complete an assessment in about an hour or so. I am just going check out my other patients first so I can spend more time in here later. Is there anything I can get you right now?"

Touching base with nursing assistants at the beginning of the shift

"Hey Travis and Denessa, how are you today? Gah, that Starbucks looks delicious. I had a white chocolate mocha yesterday. Yum. Anyways, the guy in room 73 uses the urinal but needs help or else we'll have ten total bed changes on our hands, 82 is a high fall risk who almost fell last night, and 83 will be discharged early today. Let me know when you're giving baths and I'll try to help."

When your patient or their visitors are being verbally abusive or threatening

"That is inappropriate."

"You will not speak to me in that manner."

"Do not curse at me."

"As your nurse, I am here to help you, not be disrespected."

"I am here to care for you today, it is not appropriate to speak to me in that manner."

"Hey, don't treat me like that. It's understandable that you're frustrated with everything, but you're taking it out on me. It's okay if that was your instinct, but you need to know that it's not okay to talk to me like that and we've gotta change how you're dealing with this. I'm still going to take really good care of you, even though we had this little bump in the road. Being sick sucks. I get it. And if you want to talk about it, I'm here."

"I understand that it was really frustrating to hear the doctor say what she said. I know you had a lot of hope that your family member would walk out of here, and she just told you he wouldn't. Keep in mind that we're all on the same team. We're here to support you both through this. I'm really sorry you're going through this. I'm here for you. We want to be open and honest with you about what's going on, even if it's bad news. We don't want you to be in the dark."

When your patient or their loved one is having a tough time

"I'm so sorry you're going through this."

Explaining fall prevention interventions

"So while you're in the hospital, even if you feel great, you're at a risk to fall or injure yourself. I've had some patients who felt totally normal hit the deck unexpectedly, so you can't be too careful. I know you're here for _____, but we don't want you to have to stay any longer because you got injured while recovering. We've got a few things in place to help prevent this from happening. While you're out of bed, we want you to wear these nonskid socks. Whenever you need to use the restroom, hit your call bell so we can help you. There's a lot to disconnect and keep in line when you're walking. And I'll also have this bed alarm on so if you do get confused and get out of bed without someone, it lets me know I need to come right away. If you or your loved ones see we forgot any of that, let us know. You won't be picking on us and we won't take it personally. Recovery takes a village, and we want to work together to make that happens as smoothly as possible."

Assessing your patient's understanding of and ability to use the call bell

"Before I leave I just want to make sure that you know what button to hit if you need me. Can you point to which button you need to hit if you need me? Why don't you go ahead and hit it and we'll make sure that it works?"

Index

A

abuse 54
ACLS (advanced cardiac life
    support) 135
  nurse 136
activities of daily living (ADL) 53
acute respiratory distress syndrome
    (ARDS) 172
ADL (activities of daily living) 53
admissions 46, 57, 61, 66, 72, 73, 103,
    164
  physician 57
advanced cardiac life support
    (ACLS) 135
  nurse 136
advanced practice provider 57, 60,
    62, 160, 166. *See also* nurse
    practitioner (NP); *See*
    also physician assistant (PA)
advocacy. *See also* nurse, support
  patient 22, 36
  self- 24, 34, 119
aggression 123–124, 128–129
airway 76–77, 107, 114, 134, 135, 138
allergies 56
anxiety 19, 22, 66
apologizing 103–104
application 1, 27, 32, 33, 34, 35
ARDS (acute respiratory distress
    syndrome) 172
assessment 71, 73–77, 78, 79, 102, 108,
    109, 110, 115, 123, 131, 149
  example questions 74
  neurological 115, 147
Authority Nutrition Blog 184
autopsy 134

B

basic life support (BLS) 135
bed bath 20, 22, 87, 162
bed change 9–12, 28
blood
  clot 146
  draw 21, 161
  pressure 60, 103, 114, 150
    medication. *See* medication, blood
    pressure
BLS (basic life support) 135
Board of Directors (BOD) 39
board of nursing (BON) 27, 85
  reviews 13
BOD (Board of Directors) 39
BON. *See* board of nursing (BON)
bridge program 34
Brown, Brene 190
budget
  personal 180–181
  unit 4

C

call light 21, 22, 67, 103, 105, 107, 108,
    111, 163, 164, 165
cancer 6, 56, 129, 171. *See*
    also oncologist; *See also* unit,
    oncology
cardiac arrest 131–135
cardiologist 57, 61
  pediatric 59
cardiopulmonary resuscitation
    (CPR) 132, 136, 137
career xiii, 1, 17, 27, 32, 33, 77, 191, 193
case manager 54, 68, 92
catheter 12–13, 65, 69, 90, 134, 171
certifications 4, 39

F

family members 6, 15, 27, 55, 62, 77,
    93, 107, 116, 119, 134, 137, 141
  communication 176–178
  difficult 126–130
    responses to 128
fellows 59
funeral home 134, 135
Future of Nursing 33

G

gossip 17
grade point average (GPA) 25

H

health care team xii, 21, 48, 51, 52, 54,
    56, 63–67, 68, 82, 84, 89, 113,
    160
hospice 42, 73, 129, 140, 153
hospitalist 58, 61, 132, 133
house supervisor 133, 134
human resources (HR) 35
hydration 181–182

I

ICU. *See* unit, intensive care (ICU)
inappropriate behavior
  in family members 126–130
  in patients 119–126
    responses to 120–121, 123–127, 128
infection control 80
initiative 20
injury 163–165. *See also* patient care,
    fall-risk
  prevention 163–164
Institute of Medicine (IOM) 33
insurance 54
intensivist 172
interns 57, 59
interviews 1, 34–38
  follow-up 39

peer 34
  sample questions 36, 38–39
  video 32
intuition 4, 96, 115–118
IOM (Institute of Medicine) 33

J

job search 31–40

L

labs 21, 22, 41, 65, 90, 91, 109, 114
leadership 51–70, 88
  informal 3
legal issues 54
letter of recommendation 31, 32, 34
licensed practical nurse (LPN) 85, 171
licensed vocational nurse (LVN) 85
lifestyle 175–194
  night shift 184–188
lines 76–77, 114, 115, 116, 130, 134, 162
locked-in syndrome 148
LPN (licensed practical nurse) 85, 171
LVN (licensed vocational nurse) 85

M

Magnet designation 39
magnetic resonance imaging
    (MRI) 110, 148–150, 161, 182
  techs 150
medical students 57–59
medication 2, 20, 21, 108, 114
  administration 42, 91
  blood pressure 92, 101, 112, 122
  charting 87, 103
  dispensing machine 56, 168
  dosing 56
  errors 162–163
  pain 74, 81–82, 85, 106, 108, 163
  pass 100, 110–111, 131, 162
  scheduling 102
Meister, Rustin 57–67
mentor 42–44, 49, 167